EATWELLLIVEWELL

with GLUTEN
INTOLERANCE

Visit our website at www.skyhorsepublishing.com.

10 9 8 7 6 5 4 3 2 1

Library of Congress Cataloging-in-Publication Data is available on file.

Print ISBN: 978-1-63220-446-2
Ebook ISBN: 978-1-63450-113-2

Printed in China

All the recipes in this book are free of gluten. For ingredients that typically contain gluten (such as flour, bread and cereals) we have specified that you choose a gluten-free version. For ingredients that occasionally contain gluten we have used the symbol GF so you know to check the ingredient list.

The nutritional analysis of recipes does not include any serving suggestions or garnishes.

Disclaimer

The information in this book is intended to provide people with celiac disease (with or without dermatitis herpetiformis (DH)), and people who care for them, with general advice about healthy gluten-free eating (accurate at the time of printing). This advice may not be sufficient for some people with multiple health problems or serious complications. It is not intended to replace any advice given to you by a doctor or other mainstream health professional. It is important that celiac disease and DH are diagnosed by a doctor, using standard diagnostic tests (blood samples, biopsies and assessment of your symptoms). Neither the author nor the publishers can be held responsible for claims arising from the inappropriate use or incorrect interpretation of any of the dietary advice described in this book.

Revised & Updated

EATWELLLIVEWELL

with GLUTEN
INTOLERANCE

gluten-free recipes and tips

Dr. Susanna Holt (PhD, Dietitian)

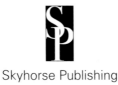

Skyhorse Publishing

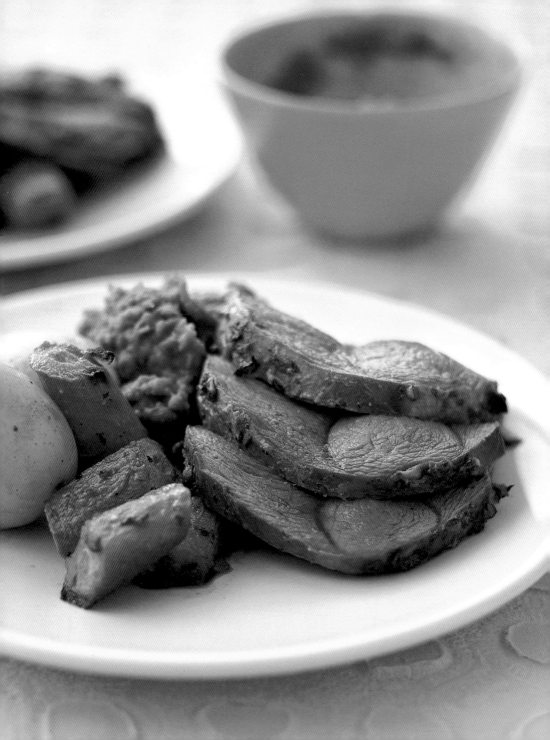

CONTENTS

LIVING WITH GLUTEN INTOLERANCE

A diagnosis of gluten intolerance no longer means the end of delicious foods. With the range of gluten-free products now available it is now much easier to follow a gluten-free diet, and with all the simple recipes in this book there are gluten-free meals for every occasion.

Who Will Benefit From This Book?

This book has been designed to provide people who need to follow a gluten-free diet, and those who cater for them, with important information about celiac disease and dermatitis herpetiformis (DH), as well as provide practical advice on healthy, gluten-free eating. If you suspect you have celiac disease or DH it is important that you consult with your doctor so the appropriate tests can be done to check if you have the condition. Once you have been diagnosed, it is recommended that you join your local celiac disease organization (for example, in the United States, the Celiac Disease Foundation). These organizations can provide invaluable support and practical advice and refer you to an expert dietitian, which is particularly beneficial in the early stages after diagnosis.

How Can This Book Help?

This book contains a broad range of tested gluten-free recipes that are relatively quick and easy to prepare. There are recipes for everyday eating and special occasions. Meals with a low glycemic index (GI), which produce a relatively small rise in the blood sugar level after they are eaten, have also been included for people who have both celiac disease and diabetes. However, these are also good choices for people without diabetes. There are plenty of recipes that will suit the whole family; so if you only have one family member who requires a gluten-free diet, you won't need to prepare different meals. Preparing gluten-free meals that the whole family can enjoy is particularly valuable if you have a child who requires a gluten-free diet because it's important to make them feel as though they're being treated like the rest of the family (it also has the other benefit of saving you time).

Why Follow A Gluten-Free Diet?

Gluten is the main protein found in wheat, barley, rye, triticale and oats. It contains an equal amount of two protein fractions called glutelin and prolamin. Gluten causes an immune reaction in people with celiac disease that damages their small intestine and impairs normal digestive processes. Currently, the only treatment for celiac disease is a lifelong gluten-free diet. Even tiny amounts of gluten should be avoided, because they can damage the small intestine. While it can be initially challenging to

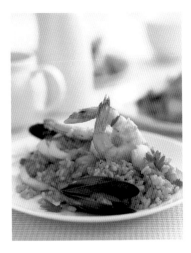

switch to a gluten-free diet and to come to terms with your condition, it's important to remember that following a gluten-free diet is less difficult than the treatment needed for many other health conditions and there are lots of resources available to help you. Due to greater availability of diagnostic tests, there has been an increase in the number of people diagnosed with celiac disease in the past fifteen years and this has led the food industry to develop an increasing range of gluten-free convenience foods. It is becoming easier to find safe gluten-free foods in supermarkets and health-food stores, or you can order them from specialist food companies over the Internet. Eating a gluten-free diet is much easier now than it was fifteen years ago, but it can still be challenging at times, particularly when you are first becoming used to the diet. However, you're not alone: there are lots of support groups, educational resources, and specialist health professionals available to help you.

What Is Celiac Disease?

Celiac (pronounced seeliac) disease is a chronic autoimmune disorder that occurs in genetically predisposed people. When people with celiac disease consume gluten, their immune system overreacts and the lining of their small intestine becomes damaged. The entire inner surface of the small intestine is lined with millions of tiny fingerlike projections called villi, which absorb water and nutrients from digested food matter as it passes through the small intestine. In people with celiac disease, the body's adverse immune reaction to gluten causes the villi to become inflamed and flattened. Without normal villi, the body is less able to absorb water and nutrients from digested food. As

Common symptoms of celiac disease include:

- excessive gas (flatulence), abdominal pain and bloating
- chronic diarrhea; pale, foul-smelling or fatty stools
- constipation
- nausea, vomiting
- weight loss
- fatigue, headaches, irritability and behavioral issues
- anemia (due to iron and/or folate deficiency)
- bone or joint pain; muscle cramps
- weakened bones (osteopenia and osteoporosis) and teeth (loss of tooth enamel and color)
- menstrual and pregnancy problems in women (missed periods; recurrent miscarriage)
- infertility in men and women
- delayed or stunted growth in infants and children
- pale sores inside the mouth, called aphthous ulcers
- itchy skin rash called dermatitis herpetiformis (DH)

the villi become progressively more damaged in people with untreated celiac disease, they can suffer from various stomach and bowel problems and nutrient deficiencies. Celiac disease is both an autoimmune disorder (because the body's immune system causes the damage) and a digestive disease (because nutrient absorption is impaired). Celiac disease can develop at any age after people start consuming gluten but many people develop the disease at around five years of age. Approximately 30 percent of people with celiac disease don't get noticeable or significant symptoms, so many people have the condition but don't know it.

What Causes Celiac Disease?

The reason why some people's immune system reacts to gluten is still being investigated, but genetic factors play a major role as the disease runs in families. You have about a one in six chance of having celiac disease if your parent, sibling, or child has it and a one in twenty chance if you have a first cousin or second-degree relative who has it. You also have an increased risk of celiac disease if you have another autoimmune condition such as Type 1 diabetes or thyroid disease. Environmental and lifestyle factors may also play a role, as celiac disease may only become active for the first time after a person experiences a period of physical or emotional stress, such as pregnancy, childbirth, surgery, intense emotional distress or a viral infection.

How Common Is Celiac Disease?

For many years, celiac disease was thought to be a relatively uncommon condition that mainly affected Caucasian people. However, recent studies have indicated that approximately 1 percent of the population in Western countries have celiac disease and many of these people remain undiagnosed. Celiac disease also appears to be more common in Africa, South America and Asia than previously believed, but the disease is most prevalent among Caucasian people of European descent. Approximately 5 percent of people with Type 1 diabetes also have celiac disease and 5–10 percent of people with Down's syndrome also have celiac disease.

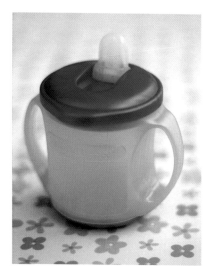

What Are The Symptoms Of Celiac Disease?

One reason why celiac disease can be difficult to diagnose is that the condition affects people differently. For example, one person might have severe abdominal pain and chronic diarrhea, while another may feel irritable and tired, and a third may not experience any noticeable symptoms at all. Both the type and onset of symptoms varies among people with celiac disease. Some people first develop symptoms as infants, whereas others don't experience symptoms until they are older. Reasons why the disease is thought to affect people differently include the length of time they were breast-fed (in general, it appears that the longer a person was breast-fed as a baby, the longer it takes for their symptoms to develop); the age a person first started eating gluten-containing foods; the amount of gluten in their diet; and differences in the body's sensitivity to gluten. The severity of symptoms experienced does not always reflect the amount of intestinal damage present, such that people with greater damage do not always have the worst symptoms. People without symptoms will still suffer intestinal damage when they eat gluten and are still at risk of developing nutrient deficiencies and other complications. The longer a person with celiac disease goes undiagnosed and untreated, the greater their chance of developing nutrient deficiencies and other complications. A prompt diagnosis is particularly important in children, because poor nutrition can cause serious developmental problems, such as growth, behavioral and learning problems.

What Health Problems Can Be Caused By Celiac Disease?

The damaged small intestine in people with untreated celiac disease has a reduced ability to absorb water and nutrients from digested food. Consequently, people with celiac disease can experience abdominal bloating and painful cramps after eating a meal

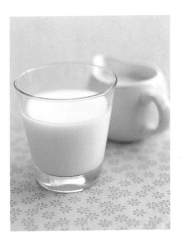

containing gluten. Unabsorbed food matter passes from the small into the large intestine, and can result in diarrhea, large smelly stools or constipation. Increased flatulence (an increased amount of smelly gas) is also a common problem because bacteria that are naturally present in the large intestine can ferment fiber and starch in the unabsorbed food matter. The impaired food absorption can also result in various nutrient deficiencies. Due to decreased iron, folate and vitamin B12 absorption, people with untreated celiac disease can develop complex anemia, which makes them feel tired and possibly also irritable and depressed. People with a severely damaged small intestine may not absorb fat, fat-soluble vitamins (vitamins A, D, E and K), zinc or protein properly, resulting in weight loss, impaired growth in children, fatigue, miscarriages, infertility and other problems. Due to decreased calcium absorption, people with celiac disease have an increased risk of osteopenia and osteoporosis (weakened bones that are more susceptible to breaking). Lactose intolerance is also common in people with undiagnosed and newly diagnosed celiac disease. This is because the damaged gut is unable to break down lactose (the sugar in cow's milk) which can lead to symptoms such as abdominal bloating and pain after dairy products are consumed. People with untreated celiac disease also have a small increased risk of esophageal and intestinal cancers, but this risk is reduced after three to five years on a gluten-free diet. A nutritious, gluten-free diet is essential for treating celiac disease and for preventing or correcting the health problems caused by the condition.

What Diseases Are Linked To Celiac Disease?

People with celiac disease have an increased risk of other autoimmune diseases including Type 1 diabetes, hypothyroidism (an under-active thyroid), systemic lupus erythematosus (Lupus), liver disease and rheumatoid arthritis. This is why it is important for people with celiac disease to have follow-up appointments with their specialist health care team members (e.g. gastroenterologist, general practitioner, dietitian) and promptly seek medical advice if any new health issues develop. After a patient has established a gluten-free diet and their health has improved, a minimum of annual physical examinations with follow-up blood tests may be required.

How Is Celiac Disease Diagnosed?

It can be difficult for doctors to diagnose celiac disease because the symptoms can be vague or similar to those of other diseases, such as irritable bowel syndrome, Crohn's disease, diverticulitis, intestinal infections, iron-deficiency anemia and chronic fatigue syndrome. Doctors may perform tests to rule out these conditions before they consider the possibility of celiac disease. Consequently, it can take months or years before a person is properly diagnosed with celiac disease. However, increased education and greater availability of diagnostic tests have made it easier for doctors to diagnose celiac disease. You should definitely inform your doctor if you have a family history of celiac disease, particularly if you also suffer from any of the associated symptoms.

Typically, testing for celiac disease starts with a simple blood test to check the blood for celiac disease antibodies. People with celiac disease who are eating gluten will have higher than normal levels of these antibodies in their blood. Therefore, it is essential that you are still eating gluten while you are being tested for celiac disease. If the blood test shows you have higher than normal levels of celiac disease antibodies, this only suggests the presence of celiac disease. An endoscopic biopsy will be required to examine your small intestine and confirm if you have celiac disease or not (or another gastrointestinal condition). You must continue eating gluten for one to three months before the procedure for the biopsy results to be accurate. Some people with dermatitis herpetiformis (DH) may require a skin biopsy instead of an endoscopic biopsy because the skin condition and skin biopsy can confirm the presence of celiac disease.

In recent times, many people have diagnosed themselves as being gluten intolerant or having celiac disease simply based on vague gastrointestinal symptoms and information they may have read on the Internet or in magazines or received from alternative health practitioners or friends. Some people may feel better when they switch to a gluten-free diet because the overall quality of their diet may have improved or they could have reduced the amount of other food components that may cause them digestive issues. However, they may not actually have celiac disease or gluten intolerance and could have another undiagnosed health condition or dietary imbalance. Therefore, it's very important that people don't self-diagnose celiac disease or gluten intolerance because they may not actually have the condition. If you think you may have one of these conditions because you regularly experience symptoms associated with these conditions or have a relative with celiac disease, discuss this with your medical doctor.

What Happens Prior To Diagnosis?

If you think that you may have celiac disease, it's important that you keep eating gluten-containing foods, such as regular wheat flour-based bread, breakfast cereals and pasta, until you have been diagnosed with celiac disease via a biopsy. If you stop eating gluten before being tested, your blood test and biopsy may be artificially negative for celiac disease even if you do have the condition (it's just not apparent at that time because you have removed gluten from your diet). If you have adopted a gluten-free diet before being tested for celiac disease, you will need to eat gluten-containing foods again for at least four to twelve weeks before undergoing the diagnostic tests (your doctor will let you know the required time period). You may suffer some symptoms during this time, but your doctor won't be able to diagnose or rule out celiac disease unless you have been eating gluten before the tests are performed. Before you have the blood test and/or the biopsy done, keep a daily diary and record the types and amounts of foods, drinks, medications and supplements you consume and document details of any symptoms or health problems you experience including how long they last for, how frequent they were and how severe they were. Give this information to your doctor at your next visit to help with a diagnosis of which health condition(s) you may have and whether you need any additional tests.

What Is Dermatitis Herpetiformis?

Dermatitis herpetiformis (DH), also known as Duhring's disease, is a non-contagious skin condition that occurs in approximately 15–25 percent of people with celiac disease

The diagnosis of celiac disease generally occurs in three steps:

1. The first step is to discuss your concerns and symptoms with your doctor.
2. If your doctor suspects celiac disease, you will need to have a blood test to check for the presence of celiac disease antibodies. These antibodies are present in higher levels in people with celiac disease.
3. If your doctor feels that there is a chance that you have celiac disease on the basis of your blood test and/or your symptoms, you will be referred to a gastroenterologist for a biopsy of your small intestine. To perform the biopsy, the gastroenterologist gradually eases a long flexible tube (endoscope) through your mouth down into your small intestine; this procedure is performed using local anesthetic to minimize discomfort and patients often report that it wasn't as uncomfortable as they were expecting it to be. A tiny instrument is passed through the endoscope to collect a small tissue sample from your small intestine. The tissue sample is then taken to a lab and examined under a microscope. If the tissue abnormalities that occur with celiac disease (inflammation and damaged villi) are found in the sample, the gastroenterologist or your doctor will inform you that you have celiac disease.

who often have no digestive symptoms. It can be misdiagnosed as eczema. DH affects people of all ages but often first appears between the ages of thirty to forty. DH results in red, raised, blistering patches that are intensely itchy and sting when scratched. These patches can flare and subside and often leave behind pale or brown areas of skin. DH can also result in a hive-like scaly rash, usually on the elbows, knees and buttocks, although it can affect any area of skin. A skin biopsy is required to diagnose DH and a strict gluten-free diet is required to control the condition possibly with some medications.

To diagnose DH, a doctor will collect a blood sample to check for celiac disease antibodies and a dermatologist (a specialist skin doctor) will take a small skin sample to check for the presence of the antibody immunoglobulin A (IgA). An intestinal biopsy may also be required if the blood and/or skin tests are not definitive for celiac disease or DH.

What's the difference between celiac disease and wheat allergy or gluten intolerance?

People with celiac disease have a permanent, lifelong intolerance to gluten and they need to maintain a gluten-free diet throughout their life in order to avoid intestinal damage and its associated complications. People with celiac disease need to avoid all sources of gluten, not only wheat. In contrast, people with wheat allergy have an immune reaction to wheat protein, which quickly results in symptoms, such as swelling around the mouth, hives, rashes and eczema. Wheat allergy usually develops in young children and disappears as they get older but, in some rare cases, it can stay with a person for life. People with wheat allergy need only avoid foods and drinks that contain the offending wheat protein. A wheat-free diet is less restrictive than a gluten-free diet. However, not all gluten-free foods are suitable for people with a wheat allergy because they may still contain some gluten-free sources of wheat protein, such as gluten-free wheat starch.

Although rare, some people have a less severe intolerance to gluten, called non-celiac gluten intolerance or gluten sensitivity. Gluten consumption causes adverse symptoms in these people, such as nausea, diarrhea, abdominal pain and bloating, but it doesn't cause the intestinal damage seen in celiac disease and they don't develop celiac disease antibodies. Since there is currently no reliable blood test for confirming gluten intolerance, people have to undergo the same blood tests and biopsies required to diagnose celiac disease as well as a gluten-free diet challenge. Gluten intolerance is considered if you are not diagnosed with a wheat allergy or celiac disease and your symptoms decrease when you eat a gluten-free diet and return when you add gluten back to your diet. The only treatment for gluten intolerance is to have a gluten-free diet, although some people with this condition can tolerate small amounts of gluten. A specialist dietitian can help you devise a suitable diet.

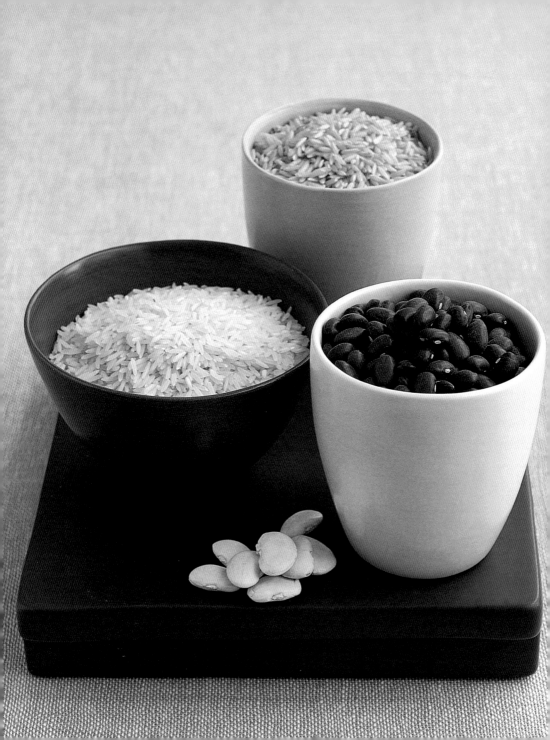

What's The Treatment For Celiac Disease?

The only treatment for celiac disease is to follow a gluten-free diet for life. Eating any gluten, no matter how small an amount, can damage the small intestine in people with celiac disease, even if they don't suffer any noticeable symptoms. Similarly, even tiny amounts of gluten can cause DH to flare up again and stop the skin from healing.

One of the best things you can do to learn about your new dietary requirements is to join your local celiac disease support organization. To find these, search the Internet or your phone directory or ask your doctor for contact information. These organizations provide useful practical information about how to best manage your condition and where to find gluten-free foods. They often offer a lot of support for its members, including supermarket tours, educational talks, regular magazines and referral to expert dietitians. It's essential that you find an experienced dietitian to help you learn how you can identify

Sources of gluten

Major sources: wheat, rye, oats*, barley, and triticale and products derived from these grains, including barley flour, bulgur/bourghul, couscous, dinkel, durum flour, einkorn wheat, emmer, farina, faro, freekah, German wheat, graham flour, kamut, oatmeal*, pilcorn, Polish wheat, rolled oats*, rye flour, semolina, spelt, wheat bran, wheat germ and foods based on wheat flour or flaked or puffed wheat (e.g. pasta, noodles, bread, breadcrumbs, breakfast cereals, brownies, cakes, cookies, crackers, croutons, donuts, muffins, rusks, pancakes, pies, pizza, flour tortillas, sauces and gravies).

Minor sources: cornstarch, dextrin, malt, malted drink powders, malt extract, malt or grain vinegar, maltodextrin, modified starch, pre-gel starch, starch, wheat starch, wheaten cornstarch, some wheat-starch based thickeners, Brewer's yeast

*Oats

Gluten contains an equal amount of two protein components called glutelin and prolamin. Prolamin is thought to be the protein fraction responsible for the damage gluten causes to people with celiac disease. Although oats contain gluten, they only contain about 5–15% of prolamins and some clinical research studies have shown that up to 4 in 5 people with celiac disease can tolerate small quantities of uncontaminated oats in their diet without symptoms or damage to their small intestine. In the USA, oats are considered to be gluten-free, but this position is not shared by health authorities in other countries because oats are often contaminated with gluten from other grains during harvesting, transport, storage, or milling and at least 1 in 5 people (20%) with celiac disease will still be damaged by uncontaminated oats. Since there is currently no simple test to determine which people will be harmed by oats, many gastroenterologists still recommend that oats should not be included in a gluten free diet. Ask your gastroenterologist for advice about whether oats are safe to include in your diet. Your gastroenterologist may recommend an intestinal biopsy before you start eating oats and 3 months after you add oats to your diet.

gluten-free foods and correct any nutritional deficiencies you may have developed while your condition was undiagnosed. If you care for someone with celiac disease, such as a child or elderly relative, then you should also attend any dietary consultations and join your local celiac organization for valuable support and education.

After starting a gluten-free diet, most people with celiac disease quickly feel much better, though for other people the symptoms can linger. In people with DH, it may take six months or more for skin problems to disappear. However, as soon as you remove gluten from your diet, your gut and skin can start to heal. The small intestine is usually completely healed and able to absorb nutrients properly within three to six months in children and younger adults and within one to two years for older adults.

What Do I Do If My Symptoms Don't Improve?

Up to 5 percent of people with celiac disease have unresponsive or refractory celiac disease where a gluten-free diet does not heal their small intestine. These people need additional follow-up with doctors and a dietitian to check for any potential sources of gluten that have been overlooked or any other causes for the intestinal damage. The most common reason for a poor response is that small amounts of gluten are still being consumed (e.g. from communion wafers, lipstick or lip balm, herbal supplements, prescription medications). Unless you become skilled at reading food labels, you may inadvertently choose gluten-containing foods when shopping. Similarly, you could make the wrong food choices when eating out. Advice from an expert dietitian is essential for helping you achieve a gluten-free diet that also meets your other nutritional needs. Contact your local celiac organization or doctor to ask if they can refer you to an expert dietitian in your area. You may need to see a dietitian frequently during the first few months after you've been diagnosed, but once you've begun mastering your new diet, you will be able to see them less often. After this, it's still worth consulting your dietitian every six to twelve months (or more often if you still have symptoms or other nutrition-related problems) for a dietary check-up. When you're prescribed medications, ask your doctor and pharmacist to check that they have given you gluten-free versions because some medications can contain gluten. You can also contact food and pharmaceutical companies directly to ask if their products contain gluten. Contact information can be found on the company websites.

What Is A Gluten-Free Diet?

A gluten-free diet means not eating foods that contain wheat (including spelt, triticale and kamut), rye, barley or oats or gluten-containing ingredients derived from these grains. Although this rules out a lot of foods, such as many types of bread, breakfast cereals, cookies and pasta, there are many gluten-free versions of these foods available at supermarkets, health-food stores and from specialist food companies. In addition to gluten-free processed foods, there are also plenty of naturally gluten-free foods available, such as fruit, vegetables, legumes, meat, fish, eggs, nuts and seeds. So, it's definitely possible to have a nutritious, balanced gluten-free diet. Rather than thinking about all of the foods you can't have, focus on enjoying all of the foods you can eat. Some people find that the diagnosis of celiac disease makes them improve the quality of their diet and their cooking skills, because they no longer rely on processed foods. It's also a great incentive to explore the huge variety of foods available, many of which you may never have eaten before, such as quinoa, buckwheat, and chickpeas.

Gluten-free options

amaranth, arrowroot, besan (chickpea flour), buckwheat, buckwheat flour, cassava, cassava flour, chia, corn/maize, cornmeal (polenta), gluten-free flour mixes, gluten-free oats, kasha, legumes, lentil flour, lotus root flour, lupin, maize cornstarch/flour (without any added wheat flour/starch), millet, modified maize starch, raw nuts, nut flours, potatoes, potato flour, potato starch, psyllium, quinoa, rice, rice bran, rice flour, sago, seeds, sorghum, soy beans, soy flour, tapioca, tapioca flour, teff, vinegar (balsamic or wine), xanthan gum

Food ingredients with no detectable gluten*

caramel color, dextrose, fructose, glucose, glucose powder, glucose syrup, maltose, wheat glucose syrup

* Even if derived from wheat.

Become A Gluten Detective: Look For Hidden Gluten In Processed Foods

A really important tool for maintaining a gluten-free diet is learning which ingredients contain gluten and thoroughly reading the information on food labels. Gluten-containing ingredients are present in many processed foods and different brands of the same product can vary in their gluten content (for example, one brand of fish sauce contains gluten, whereas another brand doesn't). An expert dietitian can help you learn how to interpret the information on food labels, and your local celiac organization can provide you with information about gluten-free products and ingredients. After a while, scanning food labels will become second nature to you and less time-consuming (initially you may need to take a list or handbook with you, if you can't remember all of the gluten-containing ingredients you need to check for). Many food companies also have lists or information about their gluten-free products that you can access on their website or by contacting the company's consumer service department (contact numbers are often listed on food labels and on websites). Some food companies refrain from adding a gluten-free label to a product, even if it really is gluten-free, because the product may not be gluten-free in the future if the company changes one of the ingredients or because they can't rule out cross-contamination (see page 18). Gluten can also be found in medicines and nutrient supplements, so ask your doctor and pharmacist to check whether there is a gluten-free version of any medication or supplement you are advised to take. The adhesive on postage stamps and envelopes may also contain gluten. So look for non-lickable stamps and envelopes or moisten stamps and envelopes with a wet sponge.

Improvements to the food labelling laws in many Western countries have made it much easier for people to find reliable gluten-free foods. All ingredients derived from gluten-containing grains must be declared in the ingredient list on food labels (for example, manufacturers have to list wheat starch rather than just starch). Products that have the words "gluten-free" on their packaging must not contain any detectable gluten. There is also a crossed-grain symbol that appears on some gluten-free foods in various countries to let you know that the product has been confirmed to be gluten-free. However, not all gluten-free foods carry this symbol and the food labelling laws differ between various countries.

Cross-contamination

When possible, always choose a product that has the words "gluten-free" written on the label because some products that you would expect to be free of gluten, such as cookies made from rice flour, may be produced in a factory that also makes gluten-containing foods, such as cookies made from wheat flour. Unless the manufacturer uses separate equipment to make the products and stores the ingredients separately, it is possible for cross-contamination to occur (for example, some wheat flour (gluten) ends up in the rice flour cookie). Some specialist food companies are well aware of the potential for cross-contamination and maintain very strict manufacturing conditions to ensure that their gluten-free products are exactly that. However, not all companies are so aware of the problems of cross-contamination. It's also important to remember that "wheat-free" products may not necessarily be free of gluten, so always check the ingredient list for any sources of gluten before purchasing wheat-free foods.

When foods are prepared in or outside the home, cross-contamination can occur when gluten-free foods/ingredients come into contact with sources of gluten. This can easily

Products that may contain gluten—always check the ingredient list

baking powder
beer, ale, lager
breading and coating mixes
breakfast cereals
brown rice syrup
cheese flavor
cheese spread
chutney
coffee whitener
compound chocolate
confectionery
tortillas
curry sauces/mixes/powder
dill pickles and gherkins
drink mixes
dry-roasted nuts

potato chips, corn chips, tortilla
  chips
frozen fries
grated cheese (pre-grated)
gravy mixes
instant dried mashed potato
lecithin
marinades
mayonnaise
mustard
pickles
processed meats (e.g. bacon, ham,
  salami, sausages)
puffed rice cakes
relish
salad dressings

sauces (e.g. fish, hoisin,
  oyster, pasta, tomato,
  soy, sichuan, tamari,
  worcestershire)
sauce/seasoning mixes
self-basting poultry
soba noodles
soup (canned and dried)
soy milk and soy yogurt
stock (ready-made, cubes or
  powder)
stuffing mixes
white pepper (flour may be added
  for extra bulk)
yeast
malt vinegars

happen when other family members or housemates do not follow a gluten-free diet. Examples of cross-contamination are listed below:

- crumbs from regular bread can be transferred to gluten-free bread in a toaster
- wheat flour residue can be transferred to gluten-free flour in a sifter
- gluten-free food is placed into an unwashed container that previously contained a gluten-containing food
- gluten-free pizza dough is prepared on a surface that contains wheat flour residue because the pizza shop prepares regular pizza bases in the same area (wheat flour can become airborne and contaminate preparation surfaces and equipment)
- gluten-free deep-fried foods (e.g. plain French fries) are cooked in the same batch of oil as breadcrumbed deep-fried foods

Your local celiac disease organization and a specialist dietitian can provide you with information about methods and equipment that can be used to avoid cross-contamination and how to choose or request safe gluten-free foods when eating out.

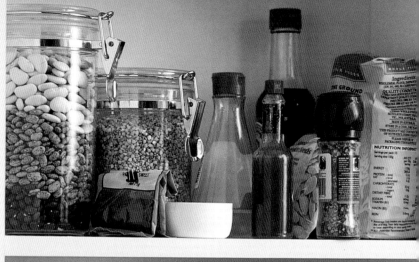
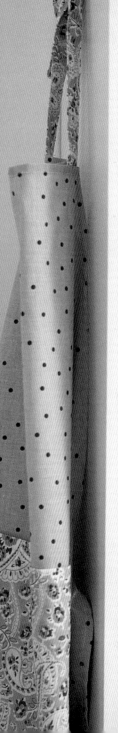
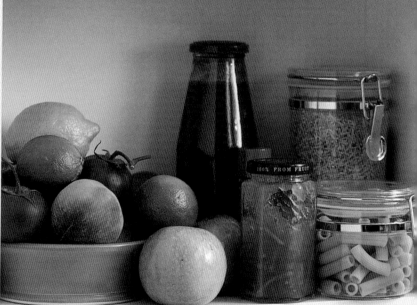
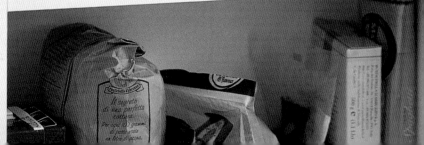

Tips For Eating A Balanced, Nutritious Gluten-Free Diet

General healthy eating guidelines for people with celiac disease are the same as those for people without these conditions—with the exception that all foods must be gluten-free and any nutrient deficiencies present after diagnosis are corrected through the sensible use of supplements and healthy eating (supplement use should be guided by your doctor and dietitian):

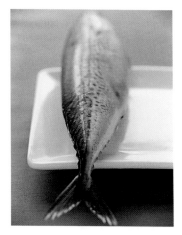

1. Eat a wide variety of nutritious foods each day

Most of the food you eat each day should be fruit, vegetables, legumes and gluten-free cereal products, such as rice and other gluten-free grains, gluten-free bread, pasta and breakfast cereals. If you also have diabetes, you should choose low-GI versions of these foods, such as basmati rice, wild rice, quinoa, sweet potato and temperate fruit. Try to eat a variety of different colored fruits and vegetables each week. Green vegetables and fresh herbs are excellent sources of folate and various antioxidants, and should be eaten daily.

2. Watch your fat intake

When the villi recover, the intestine is able to absorb more nutrients and some people will start to gain weight. This may be desirable for children and adults who have lost weight, but it's important to keep your weight within the healthy weight range. If you need to control your weight, it's important that you limit your alcohol and fat consumption. You can do this by switching to low-fat dairy products, choosing lean cuts of meat and skinless poultry, using low-fat cooking methods, and minimizing your intake of alcohol and fatty foods and added fats, such as mayonnaise, oily salad dressings, butter, cream and margarine. Aim to eat nutritious foods as snacks rather than less nutritious "junk" foods as these will help top up your body's nutrient stores. For example, choose fresh fruit or low-fat cheese on gluten-free bread instead of potato chips or confectionery.

Improve the quality of fat in your diet by making monounsaturated and omega-3 polyunsaturated fat the main fats in your diet. Unlike saturated fat, these fats help protect against heart disease and Type 2 diabetes. Increasing your omega-3 fat intake can also help reduce inflammation, which may in turn help your villi heal faster. Good sources of monounsaturated fat include avocados, olives, olive oil (preferably extra virgin), canola oil and most nuts. Good sources of omega-3 polyunsaturated fat include oily fish, such as salmon, tuna, mackerel, trout, sardines, herrings, blue eye and redfish; omega-3-enriched eggs, walnuts, linseeds (flax seeds) and canola oil. Aim to include fish in your diet 3–4 times a week. The main oils you cook with should be olive and canola oil and if you eat margarine or mayonnaise, use a lower fat variety, in moderation, based on olive or canola oil.

3. Eat moderate amounts of protein-rich foods

Red meat, poultry, eggs, liver, fish and seafood all provide good amounts of protein, iron, zinc and vitamin B12. If you have had undiagnosed celiac disease for some time, you may not have been absorbing adequate amounts of these nutrients. If so, ask your doctor to perform a blood test to check whether you are deficient in iron, folate or vitamin B12. You may initially require some nutrient supplements to build up your body's stores, particularly if you're vegetarian. Try to include rich sources of these nutrients in your diet on a regular basis (for example, red meat at least 3–4 times a week). Stir-fries are a great way to include meat, poultry, fish or seafood in your diet together with a variety of

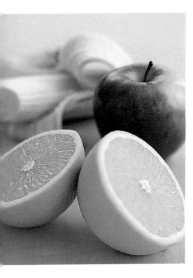

vegetables, and are delicious served with rice or gluten-free rice noodles. Vegetarian sources of protein, such as legumes, and gluten-free tofu and grain-based foods, do not provide as much iron or zinc as animal foods. If you're vegetarian, it is important to consult a dietitian for advice on how to maximize the amount of iron and zinc you absorb from your meals.

4. Regularly eat good sources of calcium

Including calcium-rich foods in your daily diet is essential for reducing the risk of osteoporosis. Dairy foods are the best sources of calcium available because lactose (milk sugar) enhances calcium absorption. Three servings of dairy products a day generally meet most people's calcium requirements (a cup of milk, 200 g (7 oz) yogurt, and a wedge of cheese). However, some people with

Recommended foods* (or gluten-free versions)	Foods to avoid

Cereal Products (grains, flours)
- Gluten-free bread, pasta, and breakfast cereals
- Porridge made from soy or rice flakes
- Gluten-free snack bars
- Noodles—rice, mung bean, buckwheat*
- Puffed rice and corn cakes*
- Gluten-free rice crackers and cookies
- Rice, millet, quinoa, buckwheat, sorghum, teff, cornmeal (cornstarch), sago, tapioca, rice bran, baby rice cereal
- Gluten-free corn tortillas and taco shells
- Rice paper, gluten-free lasagne or rice noodle sheets

- Bread containing wheat, rye, triticale, oats or barley (or any other gluten-containing ingredient)
- Muesli or breakfast cereals with gluten-containing grains, malt flavorings or malt extract
- Muesli bars, breakfast cereal snack bars
- Durum wheat pasta and wheat flour noodles (e.g. instant, udon, hokkien)
- Rolled oats, oat-based porridge, oat bran, oat meal
- Wheat bran, wheat germ, wheat meal
- Couscous
- Semolina

Fruit and Vegetables
- Fresh fruit and fruit juices
- Dried fruit*
- Fresh vegetables and fresh vegetable juice
- Plain vegetables—frozen, dried, canned and bottled*

- Some commercial fruit pie fillings
- Some snack foods with fruit fillings
- Battered vegetables and fritters
- Some brands of frozen French fries
- Textured vegetable protein
- Canned vegetables in sauce*

Legumes
- Dried legumes (soaked and freshly boiled)
- Plain, canned legumes*
- Legume flours (e.g. chickpea flour, lentil flour)

- Canned baked beans*
- Convenience vegetarian meals*

Dairy products and alternatives
- Cow's milk
- Cream, butter, sour cream
- Condensed milk*
- Coconut milk
- Gluten-free yogurts and fromage frais
- Aged cheese and soft cheese*
- Gluten-free soy milk (no malt or maltodextrin)
- Plain ice cream
- Tofu
- Rice milk

- Malted milk and some flavored milk
- Cheese spreads*
- Ice cream in a cone
- Custard* and custard powder
- Flavored ice cream*
- Some flavored yogurts and dairy desserts
- Oat milk

Beverages
- Water—tap, spring, mineral, soda, tonic
- Tea, coffee
- Soft drinks*
- Fruit juice
- Wine, liqueurs, spirits
- Carob powder and pure unsweetened cocoa powder

- Drinking chocolate and drink mixes*
- Coffee substitutes
- Lemon barley water
- Malted milk drinks
- Beer, lager, ale, stout, Guinness

Spreads and condiments
- Jam and pure fruit spreads
- Honey, golden syrup, maple syrup
- Peanut butter
- Vinegar—balsamic and wine
- Lemon juice, lime juice
- Gluten-free tamari
- Tomato paste (concentrated purée)*
- Tahini

- Yeast extract spreads – vegemite, marmite, promite
- Soy sauce*
- Commercial chutneys, relishes and pickles*
- Malt vinegar
- Commercial salad dressings* and mayonnaise*
- Many commercial sauces; different brands of the same sauce may vary in their gluten content

* Check the product's ingredient list. Individual brands may vary in their gluten content.

undiagnosed or newly diagnosed celiac disease will also be lactose intolerant due to their damaged small intestine. The lactose intolerance often disappears when the gut has healed after a period of gluten-free eating. Lactose intolerant people can choose calcium-enriched alternatives, such as gluten-free soy milk and lactose-free cow's milk, but they may also require a calcium supplement. Some people who have had long-standing untreated celiac disease and/or a low calcium intake may also require a calcium supplement to help boost their body's stores. Ask your doctor or dietitian

Products to include in a gluten-free kitchen

Pantry

gluten-free flours: white rice, potato, chickpea, soy, tapioca (store in opaque containers)

commercial gluten-free flour mixtures: plain/all-purpose, self-rising, bread mix

grains: arrowroot, quinoa, buckwheat, rice, wild rice, millet, sago, tapioca

gluten-free processed foods: bread, breakfast cereals, cookies, crackers, snack bars, pasta, and polenta

noodles: dried rice noodles, mung bean noodles

nuts and seeds: linseeds (flax seeds), chia seeds, sunflower seeds, sesame seeds and raw nuts

legumes: dried legumes and gluten-free canned varieties (e.g. chickpeas, cannellini beans, kidney beans, lentils and split peas)

fruit: gluten-free dried fruit and canned fruit

drinks: coffee and tea, plain mineral water

baking ingredients: gluten-free baking powder, baking soda, pure spices, gelatin, natural vanilla extract, xanthan gum, guar gum and psyllium fiber

sweeteners: sugar, pure confectioners' sugar, pure unsweetened cocoa powder, carob powder

milk products: UHT milk and gluten-free cow's milk alternatives, condensed milk, dried milk powder, canned coconut milk

oils: extra virgin olive oil, olive oil and canola oil snacks or serving suggestions: gluten-free taco shells and tortillas, plain popping corn, plain gluten-free poppadoms

canned fish

gluten-free sauces: tamari, fish, soy, tomato and pasta

Vegetables: onions, garlic, potatoes, sweet potatoes, pumpkin

Refrigerator

milk: cow's milk or gluten-free alternatives

fats: butter or margarine

eggs

dairy products: gluten-free cheese, yogurt, fromage frais and sour cream

spreads: pure fruit spreads, peanut butter, honey and gluten-free tahini

drinks: fruit juice, mineral water and spring water

meat: low-fat gluten-free processed meats and bacon slices

seeds and flours: ground linseeds (flax seeds), soy flour and brown rice flour (these keep for longer when stored in the refrigerator)

fresh fruit and vegetables

Freezer

gluten-free bread products: bread and breadcrumbs (fresh and dry)

gluten-free baked goods: muffins and corn tortillas,

stock: homemade gluten-free stock and meals (freeze single portions to reheat when you're too busy to cook)

gluten-free low-fat ice cream

gluten-free frozen yogurt

gluten-free yeast (this keeps better in the freezer)

frozen vegetables: spinach, peas, corn, broccoli, cauliflower and stir-fry mixtures and gluten-free oven-bake potato chips/fries for advice about whether a calcium supplement is suitable for you.

5. Include good sources of fiber in your daily diet

Relying on commercial gluten-free breads, pasta, cookies and cereals can decrease your fiber intake, because many of these commercial varieties are based on corn and rice flour which contain less fiber than wheat flour. Fiber-rich foods are important for preventing constipation and other bowel problems. Good gluten-free sources of fiber include linseed (flax) meal (you can add this to breakfast cereal, yogurt or baked goods), nuts and seeds (these can be added to salads, stir-fries and baking recipes), brown rice, buckwheat, quinoa, legumes, and fresh vegetables and fruit. And remember to drink water throughout the day—this also helps keep you regular.

6. Drink gluten-free alcohol in moderation

If you drink alcohol, enjoy it in moderation. This means 2 or fewer standard drinks for males and 1 or fewer standard drinks for females on any one day. In fact, it may be helpful to avoid alcohol entirely during the first few months after being diagnosed with celiac disease in order to help your gut heal and absorb nutrients properly. Wine, spirits and liqueurs are typically gluten-free. Beer, stout, ale, Guinness and lager should all be avoided because they contain gluten.

Make your own flour mixes

Plain (all-purpose) flour
1. Mix 6 parts rice flour with 2 parts potato flour and 1 part tapioca flour.
2. Mix 2 parts soy flour with 1 part rice flour and 1 part potato flour.
3. Use 1 part each of soy flour and potato flour; soy flour and rice flour; or soy flour and maize cornstarch.
4. Use 4 parts soy flour, 4 parts potato flour, 1 part rice flour, and 1 part glutinous rice flour.

Self-rising flour
Put 2 tablespoons potato flour into a measuring cup, then add sufficient white rice flour to bring the total volume of the mixture to 1 cup. Sift the mixture into a bowl and add 1/2 teaspoon baking soda, 1/2 teaspoon cream of tartar, and 1 teaspoon xanthan gum (or guar gum).

Baking powder
Mix together 1 part baking soda and 2 parts cream of tartar.

What Are The Challenges of Gluten-Free Baking?

Gluten provides the strength and elasticity that helps hold bakery products together. It also helps bakery products rise and obtain a light aerated texture on the inside and a crumbed texture on the surface. Consequently, gluten-free flours don't always produce

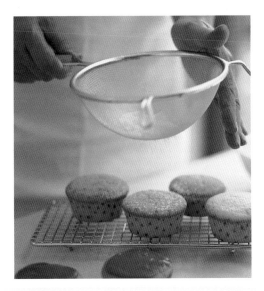

Eating well with gluten intolerance

- Keep your pantry, refrigerator and freezer well stocked with gluten-free foods, so you always have something suitable on hand when you need it.
- If you have a busy lifestyle, cook double portions of meals, so you can freeze the leftovers.
- Take suitable foods with you to work or school, to the movies, while out shopping or traveling.
- Take suitable gluten-free foods with you to parties and social events.
- Contact your local celiac organization and check the Internet and phone directory to find out about restaurants and cafés in your area that cater to people on gluten-free diets. Call restaurants ahead of time to check if their gluten-free options are suitable for you and are free from cross-contamination.
- If you're in doubt about a menu item, ask the waiter or chef about the ingredients and preparation methods or ask if a gluten-free option is available.
- If some people in your family eat regular foods and others require gluten-free foods, make sure you store the two types of foods separately to avoid cross-contamination. You may need to designate a special shelf in the pantry for gluten-free foods only, so gluten-containing foods are not grabbed by mistake. Use separate cutting boards and knives for gluten-free and regular bread, and use separate toasters (or shake out the crumbs thoroughly between toasting gluten-free bread) to make sure that gluten-free bread is not contaminated. You may also need to have separate containers of margarine, butter and spreads, so gluten-containing breadcrumbs are not eaten by family members who need to follow a gluten-free diet.
- If you have a child who requires a gluten-free diet, speak with their teachers about their condition and dietary requirements. Your child's friends and their parents should also be informed.
- If you're not certain that a food or drink does not contain gluten, do not eat it!

the same results when substituted for wheat flour. Fortunately, many people have been experimenting with gluten-free baking methods for some time, so you can benefit from the results of their experiments.

Tips For Successful Gluten-Free Baking

• In baking, a mixture of flours works best. This is why many commercial gluten-free flour mixtures contain a number of different flours.

• It's helpful to add some guar gum, xanthan gum or gluten-free pre-gel starch to gluten-free flour mixtures because they mimic the properties of gluten and help reduce crumbling in baked goods. You can get these gums from health-food stores, specialist food stores and some celiac organizations. For cakes, add 1/4 teaspoon gum per 1 cup of gluten-free flour; for breads, add 1 teaspoon gum per 1 cup of flour; for pizza crusts, add 2 teaspoons gum per 1 cup of flour. Gluten-free gluten substitute is another new ingredient that you can experiment with.

• You can make your own gluten-free flour mixture and gluten-free baking powder (see box on page 25). Sift the flours together three times before using, then substitute by weight, not by volume, when converting recipes.

• If you find the taste of regular soy flour a little unpleasant, use debittered soy flour.

• You may achieve better results by increasing the amount of baking powder in cake mixes and by adding an additional egg to gluten-free pancake batters.

• Gluten-free pastry or cookie dough is easier to work with if you refrigerate it for 30 minutes before forming into cookies.

• Applesauce can be used instead of oil in baking to add extra moisture (while reducing fat) to gluten-free waffles, cakes and pancakes (although you may need to experiment the first few times).

• Adding extra eggs, milk powder or soy flour can help to produce a less crumbly texture in gluten-free breads and cakes.

• Gluten-free bread dough often has a batter-like consistency, which means it can't be kneaded and shaped as easily as wheat-flour based bread doughs. However, you can easily make gluten-free bread rolls by using pie tins or muffin tins or you can shape molds out of aluminum foil and place them on a baking tray.

• Make sure you store gluten-free flours separately from gluten-containing flours, in labeled containers, to avoid cross-contamination. Brown rice flour and soy flour should be stored in the refrigerator, whereas other gluten-free flours can be stored in a cool dark place. For long-term storage, keep gluten-free flours in the freezer in well-sealed containers. Gluten-free yeast should also be stored in the freezer.

• Gluten-free bakery products may not keep their freshness as long as regular versions. You can freeze wrapped individual portions of gluten-free bakery goods so you can enjoy them later on.

• Using heavy-duty pans for baking, rather than aluminum ones, will help gluten-free cakes and breads cook evenly so that the center is cooked at the same time as the outside, rather than having a soggy center and a hard crust. Test your pans with a magnet—if the magnet sticks to the pan, it's fine to use. Ring-shaped pans are particularly good for cakes. To prevent the dough from sticking to the pan, grease the cooking pan before adding the dough or line it with baking paper.

• To produce a good gluten-free bakery product, you need the right ingredients and the right oven temperature. Sometimes gluten-free baked goods don't work because the oven is not working properly. You can check whether your oven is working properly by using an oven thermometer, which can be purchased from a good kitchenware shop (or over the Internet).

• Gluten-free breads can sink after being taken out of an oven if the kitchen is too humid or if the bread was left to rise too long before being placed in the oven. If you make a yeast-leavened dough that doesn't rise properly, make it again and add 1 teaspoon of vinegar or a pinch of citric acid to the water before you add the yeast.

• Make your own gluten-free dried breadcrumbs by placing gluten-free bread slices in a slow oven to dry (the bread should turn a golden color), then put the dried bread in a food processor or crush using a rolling pin. The breadcrumbs can be stored in the freezer for several months.

• Commercial gluten-free bread mixes can be used to make pizza bases (don't let the dough rise) and pancakes.

• Remember that no matter how much you experiment, some bakery products just won't work when made with gluten-free flour. However, there are plenty of other delicious gluten-free recipes you can try instead.

BREAKFAST

ROLLED RICE PORRIDGE

WHO DOESN'T LOVE PORRIDGE ON A COLD WINTER'S MORNING? USING THIS RECIPE, YOU CAN ENJOY A WARM NOURISHING PORRIDGE THAT'S FREE OF GLUTEN. TRY IT WITH A VARIETY OF TOPPINGS.

½ cup rolled rice or
   rice flakes
pure maple syrup, to serve
fresh fruit, to serve
milk, to serve

PREP TIME: 5 MINUTES
COOKING TIME: 20 MINUTES
SERVINGS: 1

Combine the rolled rice or rice flakes and 2 cups boiling water in a saucepan. Cover with a lid and simmer over medium heat for 20 minutes, or until soft and creamy. Serve topped with maple syrup, fresh fruit and milk.

HINTS:
- If you'd like a sweeter porridge, try replacing a little of the water with fruit juice. You'll need to bring it to a boil before using it.
- If you have diabetes, it's best to avoid this meal or enjoy it as an occasional treat, because it is a high-GI meal (meaning it will cause a high blood-sugar response). Use soy flakes instead of rice flakes to produce a lower GI porridge.
- Try other toppings, such as gluten-free dried fruit, rice bran, honey or brown sugar.

nutrition per serving: Energy 184 Cal; Fat 1.6 g; Saturated fat 0.4 g; Protein 4 g; Carbohydrate 39 g; Fiber 1.2 g; Cholesterol 0 mg

WHEAT-FREE MUESLI

MUESLI IS A GREAT WAY TO EAT A VARIETY OF HEALTHY FOODS IN JUST ONE BOWL. THE SEEDS AND NUTS ADD MINERALS, ANTIOXIDANTS AND FIBER, MAKING THIS MUESLI NUTRITIOUS AND SUSTAINING.

3 cups gluten-free puffed corn (nonmalted)
2 cups puffed rice
1 cup rice bran
1 cup LSA mix
½ cup roasted unsalted macadamia nuts, chopped
½ cup roasted hazelnuts, chopped
½ cup pumpkin seeds
½ cup sunflower seeds

1 cup chopped mixed dried fruit, such as dried pears, peaches and apricots
fruit juice or milk, to serve
low-fat plain yogurt, to serve

PREP TIME: 10 MINUTES
COOKING TIME: NONE
SERVINGS: 10

Put the grains, nuts, seeds and dried fruit in a large bowl and stir together thoroughly. Store in an airtight container until ready to use.

When ready to serve, top with the fruit juice or milk and the yogurt.

HINTS:
- LSA mix is a mixture of linseeds, sunflower seeds and almonds.
- To reduce the fat content of this recipe, omit the LSA mix or replace it with a little ground linseeds.
- If you would like to serve this with flavored yogurt, check the label to make sure that there are no gluten-containing ingredients.

nutrition per serving: 361 Cal; Fat 21.8 g; Saturated fat 2.4 g; Protein 8.9 g; Carbohydrate 25.9 g; Fiber 9.5 g; Cholesterol 0 mg

CITRUS SUMMER SALAD

3 ruby grapefruit
3 large oranges
1 tbsp sugar
1 cinnamon stick
1 tbsp mint, chopped
whole mint leaves, to garnish
low-fat plain yogurt, to serve

PREP TIME: 15 MINUTES
COOKING TIME: 5 MINUTES
SERVINGS: 4–6

Peel and remove the pith from the grapefruit and oranges. Carefully cut out the segments and mix together in a bowl.

Put the sugar, cinnamon stick and mint in a small saucepan with 3 tablespoons water and stir over low heat until the sugar has dissolved.

Remove the cinnamon stick and strain the mint from the syrup, then drizzle the syrup over the fruit. Garnish with fresh mint leaves and serve with yogurt.

HINTS:
- Another good combination for a citrus fruit salad is mandarins, tangelos and pomelos when they are in season. Add some pomegranate seeds for a burst of color.
- This fruit salad can be kept, covered, in the refrigerator for up to 2 days and the flavor will improve over time.
- If you take prescription medication, check whether you can still eat grapefruit while taking this medication (ask your pharmacist or check the information sheet inside the medication pack). Grapefruit contains a compound that can interfere with the metabolism of certain medications. If you do take a prescription drug, you can simply swap the grapefruit with mandarins, tangelos or any other fruit of your choice.
- If you use flavored yogurt instead of plain, check the ingredient list to ensure the yogurt is free of gluten.

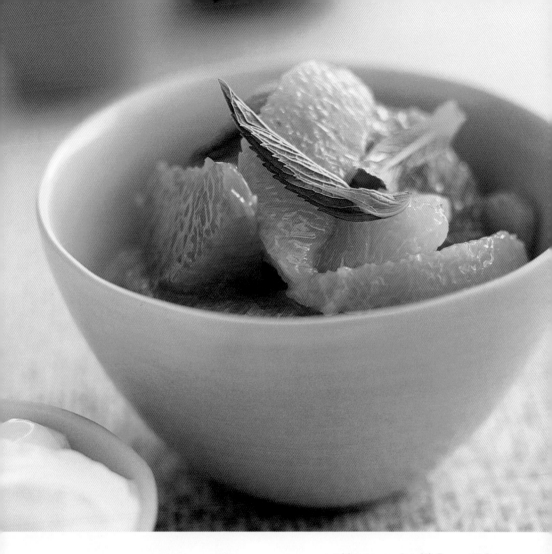

THIS REFRESHING CITRUS FRUIT SALAD WILL GIVE YOU A BOOST OF ANTIOXIDANTS AND IS A GREAT CHOICE WHEN YOU WANT A LIGHT BUT HEALTHY MEAL. TOP IT WITH SOME GLUTEN-FREE YOGURT FOR EXTRA PROTEIN AND CALCIUM. IT'S ALSO GOOD AS A SNACK.

nutrition per serving: (6): Energy 75 Cal
Fat 0.3 g
Saturated fat 0 g
Protein 2 g
Carbohydrate 15.6 g
Fiber 2.8 g
Cholesterol 0 mg

PANCAKES

YOU DON'T NEED TO MISS OUT ON DELICIOUS FOOD JUST BECAUSE YOU'RE ON A GLUTEN-FREE DIET. BY CHOOSING THE RIGHT INGREDIENTS, YOU CAN MAKE GLUTEN-FREE VERSIONS OF MANY POPULAR RECIPES, LIKE THESE PANCAKES.

1¼ cups gluten-free all-purpose flour
2 tsp gluten-free baking powder
1 egg
1 tbsp canola or olive oil
mixed berries, to serve
pure maple syrup, to serve

PREP TIME: 10 MINUTES
COOKING TIME: 20 MINUTES
MAKES 10

Sift the flour and baking powder into a bowl and make a well in the center. Mix together the egg, oil and 1¼ cups water, then add to the well in the dry ingredients. Stir until the batter is smooth and reaches the consistency of thin cream, adding up to another 3 tablespoons water if necessary. Strain the batter into a vessel with a pouring lip.

Lightly brush an 8 in frying pan with oil and heat over medium heat. Pour in just enough mixture to thinly cover the bottom of the pan. When the top of the pancake starts to set, use a spatula to turn it over. After browning the second side, transfer to a plate. Repeat with the remaining pancake batter, greasing the pan between each batch. Serve with berries and maple syrup.

HINTS:
- The pancake batter can be made the day before and stored in a covered container in the refrigerator—a great time saver in the morning.
- Pure maple syrup is concentrated from the sap of the maple tree. Do not confuse it with the cheaper maple-flavored syrup, which is artificially colored and flavored and has a much higher GI value (so it will cause a high blood-sugar response).
- These pancakes go well with many different toppings, for example, pure fruit jam, lemon juice with sugar, and even gluten-free chocolate hazelnut spread.

nutrition per pancake: Energy 97 Cal; Fat 2.7 g; Saturated fat 0.4 g; Protein 0.9 g; Carbohydrate 17 g; Fiber 0.3 g; Cholesterol 19 mg

BUCKWHEAT PANCAKES

HERE'S ANOTHER DELICIOUS GLUTEN-FREE VERSION OF PANCAKES THAT THE WHOLE FAMILY WILL ENJOY. USE WHOLE KERNEL (GROAT) BUCKWHEAT FLOUR FOR EXTRA NUTRIENTS (FIBER, PROTEIN, VITAMINS AND MINERALS).

1 cup buckwheat flour
1 egg
pure maple syrup, to serve

PREP TIME: 10 MINUTES
COOKING TIME: 20 MINUTES
MAKES 16–20

Sift the flour into a bowl and make a well in the center. In a separate bowl mix the egg with ¾ cup water, then pour into the well in the dry ingredients. Beat with a wooden spoon until the batter is combined and smooth. Pour the batter into a vessel with a pouring lip.

Brush a 8 in frying pan with oil and heat over medium heat. Pour in just enough batter to thinly cover the bottom of the pan.

When the top of the pancake starts to set, turn it over with a spatula. After browning the second side, transfer to a plate. Repeat with the remaining pancake batter, greasing the pan between batches. Serve with a drizzle of maple syrup.

HINTS:
• These pancakes are also delicious served with other toppings, such as pure fruit jam, fresh berries and gluten-free yogurt—just to name a few.
• If you're watching your weight, use spray oil to grease the pan.
• If some members of your family eat gluten, make sure to store the gluten-free and gluten-containing products (especially flour) separately to avoid cross-contamination.

nutrition per pancake (20): Energy 28 Cal; Fat 0.7 g; Saturated fat 0.2 g; Protein 1.2 g; Carbohydrate 4.1 g; Fiber 0.7 g; Cholesterol 9 mg

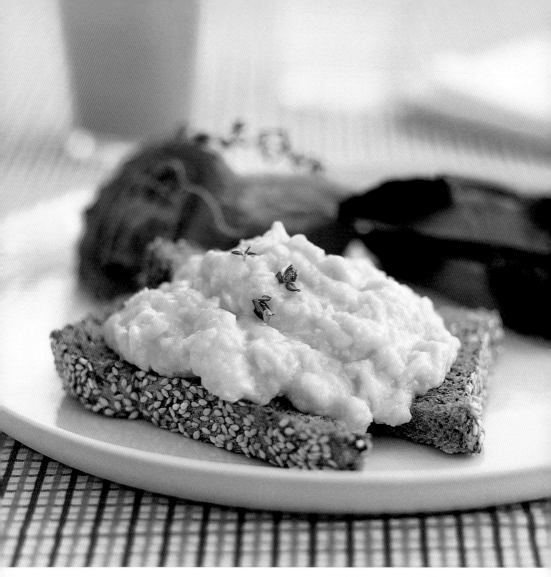

SCRAMBLED EGGS ARE ONE OF
THE ALL-TIME CLASSIC BREAKFAST
MEALS. ADDING GRILLED
MUSHROOMS AND TOMATOES
MAKES THEM EVEN MORE
DELICIOUS AND NUTRITIOUS.

nutrition per serving: Energy 550 Cal
Fat 29.3 g
Saturated fat 6.8 g
Protein 30.5 g
Carbohydrate 41.4 g
Fiber 7.1 g
Cholesterol 563 mg

SCRAMBLED EGGS WITH GRILLED TOMATOES AND MUSHROOMS

4 field mushrooms

2 vine-ripened tomatoes, halved

canola or olive oil spray

2 tsp thyme, plus extra to garnish

6 eggs

1 tbsp reduced-fat milk

2 tbsp reduced-fat canola or olive oil margarine

4 slices of gluten-free bread, toasted

PREP TIME: 5 MINUTES

COOKING TIME: 10 MINUTES

SERVINGS: 2

Put the mushrooms and tomatoes, cut side up, under a preheated broiler, then spray with oil and scatter with the thyme leaves. Cook for 3–5 minutes, or until warmed.

Meanwhile, break the eggs into a bowl, add the milk and season well with salt and freshly ground black pepper. Whisk gently with a fork until well combined.

Melt half the margarine in a small non-stick saucepan or frying pan over low heat. Add the eggs, then stir constantly with a wooden spoon. Do not turn up the heat—scrambling must be done slowly and gently. When most of the egg has set, add the remaining margarine and remove the pan from the heat. There should be enough heat left in the pan to finish cooking the eggs and melt the margarine. Serve immediately on toast. Arrange the tomatoes and mushrooms on the side. Garnish with extra thyme leaves.

HINTS:
- For the best results, use fresh eggs when scrambling. To check whether an egg is fresh, put it in a bowl of cold water. If the egg sinks on its side it is fresh; if it floats on its end it is stale. If it is somewhere between the two it is not perfectly fresh but still good enough to use for scrambled eggs.
- If some members of your family eat gluten-containing bread, make sure to use separate toasters or shake out the crumbs before each use.

CRUMPETS

MANY PEOPLE THINK THAT A GLUTEN-FREE DIET MEANS GIVING UP BREAD AND BAKERY PRODUCTS COMPLETELY. FORTUNATELY, THAT'S NOT TRUE. IF YOU LOVE CRUMPETS, GIVE THIS RECIPE A TRY.

3 cups gluten-free self-rising flour
1 tbsp sugar
1 tsp salt
2 tsp dried yeast GF
1¾ cups lukewarm milk
½ tsp baking soda
butter, to serve
strawberry jam GF**, to serve**

PREP TIME: 15 MINUTES +
1¼ HOURS STANDING
COOKING TIME: 45 MINUTES
MAKES 10

Combine the flour, sugar, salt and yeast in a large bowl. Pour in the milk and whisk well to combine. Cover and set aside in a warm place for 1 hour, or until doubled in size.

Use a spoon to beat the mixture until it deflates. Combine 4 tablespoons lukewarm water and the bicarbonate of soda in a small bowl, then whisk into the batter until smooth. Set aside for 15 minutes.

Brush a large heavy-based non-stick frying pan with oil and heat over medium heat. Brush four 3¾ x ¾ in crumpet rings with oil, then place in the pan and reduce the heat to low. Pour enough batter into each crumpet ring to fill to three-quarters full. Cook for 12–15 minutes, or until large bubbles come to the surface, the base is golden and the top is set (if the bubbles don't pop you can use a skewer to pierce the holes). Cover the pan and cook for a further 2–3 minutes. Use a sharp knife to carefully loosen the crumpets and remove from the rings. Put the crumpets on a wire rack. Wash the crumpet rings and regrease. Repeat with the remaining batter. Serve with butter and fruit jam.

HINTS:
- You can buy crumpet rings from some supermarkets and kitchenware shops.
- Each brand of commercial gluten-free flour mixture varies in the amount of different flours it contains. This means that some brands may work better with certain recipes than others, so be prepared to experiment. Check the flour's packaging to see if there is any information about the types of recipes that the flour mixture suits best.
- Gluten-free yeast should be stored in the freezer.

nutrition per serving: Energy 202 Cal; Fat 2.8 g; Saturated fat 1.2 g; Protein 3.7 g; Carbohydrate 39 g; Fiber 3.8 g; Cholesterol 6 mg

WAFFLES

HERE'S ANOTHER SURPRISE—GLUTEN-FREE WAFFLES. YOU WILL NEED A
WAFFLE IRON TO MAKE THESE AND YOU MAY NEED TO TRY DIFFERENT BRANDS
OF GLUTEN-FREE FLOUR TO FIND THE ONE THAT GIVES THE BEST RESULT.

**2 cups soy-containing,
gluten-free self-rising flour**
3 tbsp sugar
1¼ cups milk
2 eggs
¼ cup butter, melted, cooled
butter, to serve
strawberry jam GF, to serve

PREP TIME: 10 MINUTES +
15 MINUTES RESTING
COOKING TIME: 30 MINUTES
MAKES 6

To make the batter, sift the flour into a large bowl, stir in the sugar, then make a well in the center. In a separate bowl, whisk the milk and eggs together. Pour the milk mixture into the well in the dry ingredients and whisk until smooth. Whisk in the melted butter. Set the batter aside to rest for 10–15 minutes.

Preheat a waffle maker. Pour ⅓-cupfuls of the batter into the waffle maker and cook following the waffle maker's instructions. Transfer to a wire rack and repeat with the remaining batter, allowing the waffle maker to reheat between waffles. Serve the waffles with strawberry jam.

HINTS:
- It's important to use a gluten-free flour that contains soy flour when making these waffles. Soy flour acts more like gluten flour so gives a better result in some recipes. Check the ingredients list of the flour.
- You can make these waffles with rice drink or gluten-free soy milk, if you can't use cow's milk.
- These waffles are great with a variety of toppings, such as pure maple syrup, golden syrup, honey or fruit jam. If you buy jam, check the label to ensure it is free of gluten.

nutrition per serving: Energy 309 Cal; Fat 12.5 g; Saturated fat 5.3 g; Protein 7.2 g; Carbohydrate 40 g; Fiber 2.5 g; Cholesterol 82 mg

POACHED EGGS WITH SPINACH AND GARLIC YOGURT DRESSING

DRESSING
½ cup low-fat plain yogurt
1 small garlic clove, crushed
1 tbsp snipped chives

6 cups baby English spinach leaves
2 tbsp butter
4 tomatoes, halved

1 tbsp white vinegar
8 eggs
8 thick slices of gluten-free bread, toasted

PREP TIME: 10 MINUTES
COOKING TIME: 15 MINUTES
SERVINGS: 4

To make the dressing, mix together the yogurt, garlic and chives.

Wash the spinach and put it in a large saucepan with just the little water that is left clinging to the leaves. Cover the pan and cook over low heat for 3–4 minutes, or until the spinach has wilted. Add the butter, then season with salt and freshly ground black pepper and toss together. Remove the pan from the heat and keep warm.

Put the tomatoes, cut side up, under a preheated broiler and cook for 3–5 minutes, or until softened and warm.

Fill a deep frying pan three-quarters full with cold water and add the vinegar and some salt to stop the egg whites spreading. Bring the water to a gentle simmer. Gently break an egg into a small bowl, then carefully slide the egg into the water, then repeat with the remaining eggs. Reduce the heat so that the water barely moves. Cook for 1–2 minutes, or until the eggs are just set. Remove with a spatula. Drain on paper towels.

Top each slice of toast with some spinach, an egg and some dressing. Serve with the grilled tomato halves on the side.

HINTS:
- Don't use malt vinegar in the poaching water—it contains gluten.
- Avoid cross-contamination by using separate toasters for gluten-containing and glutenfree bread. Alternatively, shake out the crumbs before each use.

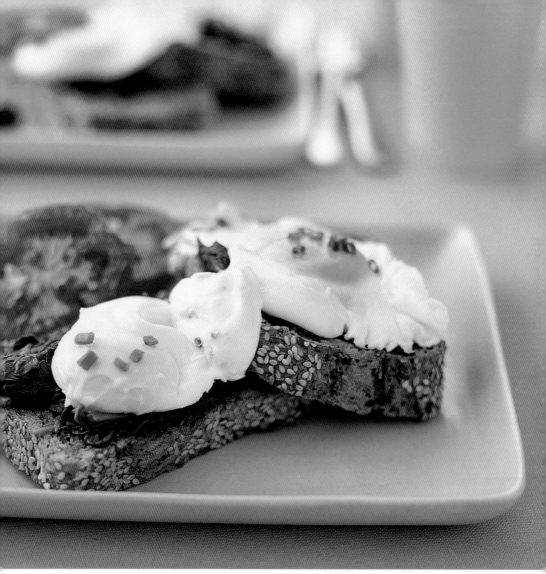

THIS NUTRITIOUS MEAL IS A GREAT CHOICE FOR CHILDREN AND ADULTS WHO HAVE HAD LONG-STANDING UNTREATED CELIAC DISEASE BECAUSE IT PROVIDES SO MANY IMPORTANT NUTRIENTS, SUCH AS IRON, ZINC, FOLATE AND VITAMINS A, B12 AND D.

nutrition per serving: Energy 422 Cal
Fat 16.1 g
Saturated fat 5.4 g
Protein 26.1 g
Carbohydrate 42.5 g
Fiber 8.3 g
Cholesterol 386 mg

41

HOMEMADE BAKED BEANS

SOME BRANDS OF COMMERCIAL BAKED BEANS ARE NOT GLUTEN-FREE, SO STAY ON THE SAFE SIDE AND MAKE YOUR OWN. HOMEMADE BAKED BEANS ARE A GREAT CHOICE FOR PEOPLE WITH DIABETES BECAUSE THEY ARE LOW GI.

3 cups dried soybeans
15 oz canned diced tomatoes
1 cup vegetable stock (Basics)
1 bay leaf
2 tbsp chopped parsley
pinch of dried thyme
1 tbsp canola or olive oil

PREP TIME: 5 MINUTES
COOKING TIME: 4 HOURS 40 MINUTES
SERVINGS: 6

Cook the soybeans in plenty of water for about 4 hours, or until tender. Drain. Preheat the oven to 350°F.

Put the soybeans in a casserole dish and add the canned tomatoes, stock, herbs and oil. Bake, covered, for 40 minutes. Check the consistency of the sauce. If you want a thicker consistency, remove the lid of the casserole dish and cook for a further 10–15 minutes, or until reduced to the desired consistency.

HINTS:
- Some brands of stock (ready-to-use, cubes and powder) are not gluten free, so check the ingredient list if you are using a commercial brand.
- When serving baked beans for breakfast, serve with toasted gluten-free bread. Baked beans can also be served as a light meal with rice or gluten-free corn tortillas.

nutrition per serving: Energy 358 Cal; Fat 21.7 g; Saturated fat 3.1 g; Protein 29.6 g; Carbohydrate 9.9 g; Fiber 19.7 g; Cholesterol 3 mg

EGGS EN COCOTTE

You don't necessarily need to cook separate meals for different family members if only one of them needs a gluten-free diet. Recipes like this one can feed the whole family.

1 tbsp olive oil
1 garlic clove, crushed
3 vine-ripened tomatoes (about 10½ oz), peeled, seeded and chopped
½ tsp olive oil, extra
4 eggs
2 tbsp snipped chives
4 slices of thick gluten-free bread
2 tbsp butter

Prep time: 15 minutes
Cooking time: 30 minutes
Servings: 4

Preheat the oven to 350°F. To make the tomato sauce, heat the oil in a heavy-based frying pan. Add the garlic and cook for 30 seconds. Add the tomato and season with salt and freshly ground black pepper. Cook over medium heat for 15 minutes, or until thickened.

Grease four ½ cup ramekins with the extra olive oil, then carefully break 1 egg into each, trying not to break the yolk. Pour the tomato sauce evenly around the outside of each egg, so the yolk is still visible. Sprinkle with chives and season lightly with salt and freshly ground black pepper.

Place the ramekins in a deep baking dish and pour in enough hot water to come halfway up the outside of the ramekins. Bake for about 10–12 minutes, or until the egg white is set. Toast the bread and lightly spread the slices with the butter. Serve immediately with the cooked eggs.

HINTS:
- If you are serving this to children, cut the toast into fingers to dip into the egg.
- People with celiac disease have to be careful to avoid even small amounts of gluten, so make sure you use separate toasters for gluten-free and gluten-containing breads to avoid cross-contamination; alternatively, shake out the crumbs before each use.

nutrition per serving: Energy 274 Cal; Fat 13.5 g; Saturated fat 4.4 g; Protein 10.6 g; Carbohydrate 26.7 g; Fiber 1.6 g; Cholesterol 200 mg

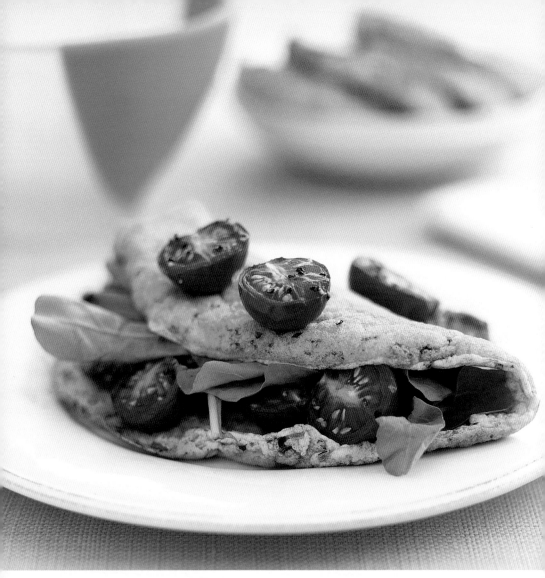

HERE'S ANOTHER EGG-BASED
DISH THAT CAN BE ENJOYED
ANYTIME. THIS RECIPE SHOWS
YOU HOW EASY IT IS TO SLIP
EXTRA VEGETABLES AND
HERBS INTO YOUR DIET TO ADD
NUTRIENTS WITHOUT ADDING
TOO MANY EXTRA CALORIES.

nutrition per serving: Energy 340 Cal

Fat 14.2 g

Saturated fat 4.4 g

Protein 26.6 g

Carbohydrate 25.3 g

Fiber 2.3 g

Cholesterol 384 mg

44

HERB OMELETTE WITH TOMATOES

9 oz red or yellow cherry tomatoes, halved
4 eggs, lightly beaten
1 handful chopped mixed herbs
  (e.g. parsley, chives, oregano)
2 egg whites
3 tbsp grated low-fat cheddar cheese ^{GF}
1 handful baby arugula leaves
2 slices of gluten-free bread, toasted

PREP TIME: 15 MINUTES
COOKING TIME: 20 MINUTES
SERVINGS: 2

Preheat the oven to 350°F. Line a baking tray with baking paper. Place the tomatoes, cut side up, on the prepared tray. Season well with salt and freshly ground black pepper. Bake for 15 minutes, or until softened. Reserve about one-third of the tomatoes for garnish.

Whisk together the whole eggs and mixed herbs in a bowl. Beat the egg whites in a small bowl with electric beaters until soft peaks form. Gently whisk the egg whites into the egg and herb mixture.

Preheat a broiler to medium heat. Heat an 8 1/2 in omelette pan or frying pan and lightly brush with oil. Pour in half of the egg mixture and leave for 1–2 minutes, or until lightly browned underneath.

Scatter half the cheese over the egg mixture and place the pan under the broiler for 1 minute, or until the egg is set and the cheese is melted. Top with half of the remaining tomatoes and half of the arugula. Fold the omelette in half and carefully slide from the pan onto a plate. Scatter half of the reserved tomatoes over the omelette.

Gently re-whisk the remaining egg mixture, then cook a second omelette in the same way as the first. Serve with the toast.

HINTS:
• If you buy ready-to-use grated cheese, check the ingredient list for any sources of gluten. Flour may be added to stop the cheese from sticking.
• Choose eggs enriched with omega-3 essential fatty acids to get more good fats in your diet. These are available in most supermarkets.
• Use baby spinach instead of baby arugula, if you prefer.
• Even small amounts of gluten can be damaging to a person with celiac disease. Avoid cross-contamination by using separate toasters for gluten-containing and gluten-free bread or, at the very least, shake out the crumbs between each use.

45

DRIED FRUIT COMPOTE

THIS FRUITY DISH CAN BE ENJOYED ON ITS OWN OR USED AS A TOPPING FOR GLUTEN-FREE PORRIDGE, YOGURT OR BREAKFAST CEREAL. IT'S DELICIOUS EITHER COLD OR WARM AND IS LOADED WITH FIBER AND ANTIOXIDANTS.

3 cups dried fruit salad mixture (dried peaches, prunes, pears, apricots, apples and nectarines)
2 cups orange juice
1 tsp brown sugar
1–2 star anise
1 vanilla bean, halved lengthways
low-fat plain yogurt, to serve

PREP TIME: 10 MINUTES
COOKING TIME: 15 MINUTES
SERVINGS: 4

Put the dried fruit salad mixture in a saucepan. Add the orange juice, sugar, star anise and vanilla bean. Bring slowly to a boil, then reduce the heat, cover and leave to simmer, stirring occasionally, for 15 minutes, or until the fruit is plump and juicy.

Discard the star anise and vanilla bean. Serve the fruit drizzled with the cooking syrup. Add a dollop of yogurt to serve.

HINTS:
- For a slightly different flavor, use a cinnamon stick and 2 cloves instead of the star anise and vanilla bean.
- If you prefer flavored yogurt over plain, make sure to check the label to ensure the yogurt is free of gluten.

nutrition per serving: Energy 295 Cal; Fat 0.5 g; Saturated fat 0 g; Protein 3.8 g; Carbohydrate 70.8 g; Fiber 7.9 g; Cholesterol 0 mg

FRESH FRUIT QUINOA

THIS IS A GOOD RECIPE TO TRY IF YOU'RE UNFAMILIAR WITH QUINOA, A TINY GLUTEN-FREE GRAIN. QUINOA TAKES LITTLE TIME TO PREPARE AND HAS A LIGHT TEXTURE AND MILD TASTE.

1 cup organic quinoa
2 cups unsweetened apple and cranberry juice
1 cinnamon stick
2 tsp grated orange zest
2 fresh figs, chopped
2 peaches or nectarines
1⅓ cups strawberries, hulled and chopped
low-fat plain yogurt, to serve
mint leaves, to garnish

PREP TIME: 10 MINUTES
COOKING TIME: 15 MINUTES
SERVINGS: 4—6

Rinse the quinoa under cold running water and drain. Put the quinoa, juice and cinnamon stick in a saucepan.

Bring to a boil, cover and simmer for 10–15 minutes, or until all the liquid has been absorbed and the quinoa is translucent and the spiral germ ring is visible. Remove the cinnamon stick. Cover and set aside to firm up and cool a little.

Fold in the orange zest and half of the chopped fruit. Spoon the mixture into four bowls and sprinkle with the remaining fruit. Serve with a generous dollop of the yogurt. Garnish with fresh mint leaves and serve immediately.

HINT:
- Quinoa is pronounced "keen-wa." It has been cultivated in the South American Andes for 500 years. It is now grown in and exported from Peru and the United States. Quinoa can be used as a substitute for couscous and can be found in health-food stores and in the health-food section of supermarkets.
- If you want to serve a flavored yogurt with this recipe, check the label to ensure the yogurt is free of gluten.

nutrition per serving: (6): Energy 176 Cal; Fat 1.8 g; Saturated fat 0.2 g; Protein 5.1 g; Carbohydrate 32.4 g; Fiber 3.8 g; Cholesterol 0 mg

ITALIAN-STYLE BREAKFAST TOASTS

4 **Roma (plum) tomatoes, halved**
2 **large field mushrooms, halved**
canola or olive oil spray
8 **slices of low-fat bacon** GF
⅔ **cup plain cottage cheese**
2 **tbsp chopped flat-leaf (Italian) parsley**
1 **tbsp snipped chives**
4 **slices of gluten-free bread, toasted**
balsamic vinegar, to drizzle

PREP TIME: 15 MINUTES
COOKING TIME: 10 MINUTES
SERVINGS: 4

Preheat the broiler. Place the tomatoes, cut side up, and the mushrooms on a large baking tray. Lightly spray with the oil. Season well with black pepper. Pat the bacon dry with paper towels and place on the tray. Broil the tomatoes, mushrooms and bacon for 5–8 minutes, or until cooked. Turn the bacon slices once and remove them as they cook and become crisp.

Combine the cottage cheese, parsley and chives. Spread thickly over the toasted bread. Arrange the tomatoes, mushrooms and bacon over the top. Drizzle with a little balsamic vinegar, then serve while hot.

HINTS:
• Gluten can be found in the most unlikely of sources, such as bacon. Check the label on the packet to ensure you buy gluten-free bacon.
• This recipe will work best with a gluten-free bread that toasts well. You may need to experiment with different types before you find the bread that toasts the best.
• Remember to keep gluten-free and regular bread separate if you live in a household where not everyone eats gluten-free foods. You will need to prepare the different types of bread on different cutting boards and with separate utensils to avoid crosscontamination. You may even need separate toasters or you will need to thoroughly shake out the crumbs from the toaster before you toast your gluten-free bread. Alternatively, some organizations helping people with celiac disease sell protective bags to cover bread while it is being toasted. It is a great invention that makes it easier to avoid cross-contamination if you don't have separate toasters.

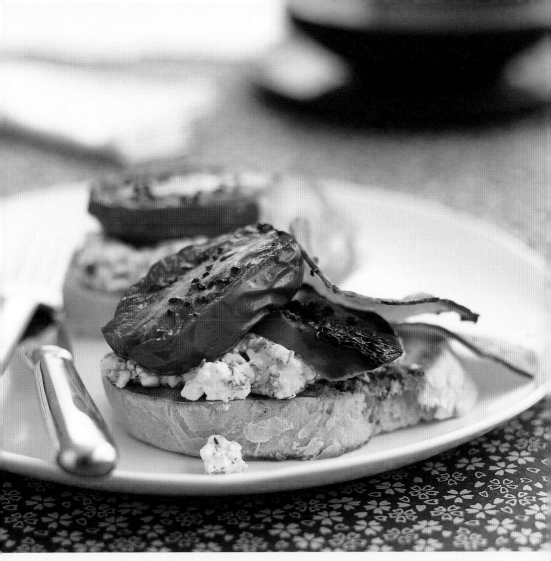

BY USING LOW-FAT BACON IN THIS
MEAL, YOU CAN STILL ENJOY A
GREAT BACON FLAVOR WITHOUT
TOO MUCH FAT. THE VARIETY OF
FOODS (MEAT, VEGETABLES, DAIRY
AND GRAIN PRODUCTS) PROVIDES
FLAVOR AND GOOD AMOUNTS OF
MANY VITAL NUTRIENTS.

nutrition per serving: Energy 278 Cal

Fat 5 g

Saturated fat 2.5 g

Protein 21.1 g

Carbohydrate 25.4 g

Fiber 1.7 g

Cholesterol 29 mg

SNACKS, LIGHT MEALS AND SIDES

PUFFED CORN SNACK MIX

**12 cups gluten-free puffed corn breakfast
 cereal**
14 oz dried fruit and raw nut mixture
1 cup rice bran
1 cup flaked coconut, toasted
4 tbsp pumpkin seeds
¾ cup honey

PREP TIME: 10 MINUTES
COOKING TIME: 20 MINUTES
SERVINGS: 20

Preheat the oven to 350°F. Line four baking trays with baking paper. Place the puffed corn, dried fruit and nut mixture, bran, flaked coconut and pumpkin seeds in a large bowl and mix together well.

Heat the honey in a saucepan over low heat for 3 minutes, or until it thins to a pouring consistency. Pour over the puffed corn mixture and stir until all the dry ingredients are well coated with the honey.

Spread the mixture on the lined baking trays in a single layer and bake for 15 minutes, or until golden, turning the cereal several times during cooking. Cool completely before storing in an airtight container in a cool, dark place.

HINTS:
* If you want to lower the fat content, leave out the flaked coconut.
* Pumpkin seeds are available at most supermarkets and health-food stores, and they make a tasty snack.

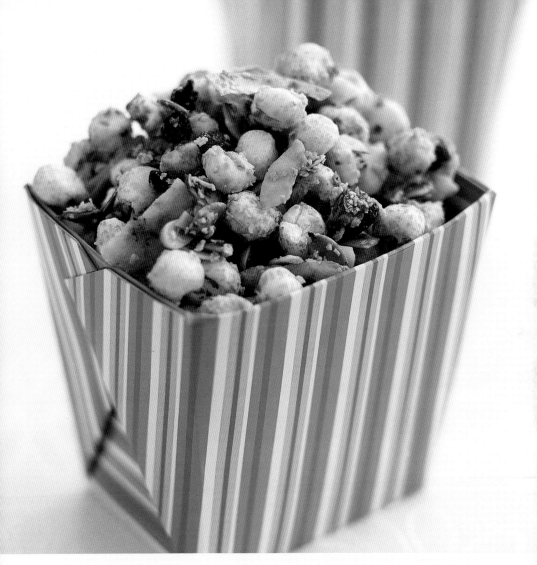

MANY COMMERCIAL SNACK FOODS
CONTAIN GLUTEN, SO MAKING YOUR
OWN GLUTEN-FREE SNACKS MAKES
SENSE. YOU CAN EASILY PACK A
SMALL CONTAINER OF THIS MIX TO
TAKE WITH YOU TO WORK, SCHOOL
OR WHEN TRAVELLING.

nutrition per serving: Energy 269 Cal
Fat 15.8 g
Saturated fat 2.1 g
Protein 20 g
Carbohydrate 7.9 g
Fiber 12.1 g
Cholesterol 3 mg

TAMARI NUT MIX

THIS YUMMY NUT AND SEED MIX IS GREAT FOR PEOPLE WHO LOVE SAVORY SNACKS AND IS PERFECT FOR WHEN YOU ENTERTAIN. THE NUTS AND SEEDS ADD A LOT OF FAT (MOSTLY UNSATURATED), SO ENJOY IN MODERATION.

1¾ cups mixed raw unsalted nuts
   (almonds, Brazil nuts, peanuts, walnuts)
¾ cup pumpkin seeds
1 cup sunflower seeds
¾ cup raw unsalted cashew nuts
scant 1 cup raw unsalted macadamia nuts
½ cup tamari

PREP TIME: 10 MINUTES +
  10 MINUTES STANDING
COOKING TIME: 25 MINUTES
MAKES 4 CUPS
SERVINGS: 12

Preheat the oven to 275°F. You will need two large baking trays.

Place the mixed nuts, pumpkin seeds, sunflower seeds, cashew nuts and macadamia nuts in a large bowl. Pour the tamari over the nuts and seeds, then toss together well, coating them evenly. Set aside for 10 minutes.

Spread the nut and seed mixture evenly over the baking trays and bake for 20–25 minutes, or until dry-roasted as desired. Cool completely.

HINTS:
- Dry-roasted nuts may be dusted with wheat flour, so make sure you use raw, gluten-free nuts in this recipe.
- Tamari is a fermented soy product similar to soy sauce. It is made with 100 percent whole soybeans, so it is much stronger than regular soy sauce and you don't need to use as much. Tamari is traditionally free of wheat but check the label to ensure it is also free of gluten.
- Don't worry if the nut mixture does not seem crisp when you take it out of the oven. It won't crisp to its full potential until it is cooled. Store in an airtight container away from direct sunlight for up to 2 weeks. If the nut mixture becomes soft, lay the nuts on a baking tray and bake in a 300°F oven for 5–10 minutes.

nutrition per serving: Energy 385 Cal; Fat 34.3 g; Saturated fat 4.5 g; Protein 12.2 g; Carbohydrate 5.7 g; Fiber 5.1 g; Cholesterol 0 mg

HUMMUS

NO WONDER HUMMUS IS POPULAR! IT'S SO DELICIOUS AND VERSATILE. IT
CAN BE SERVED AS A DIP WITH FRESH VEGETABLE STICKS AND GLUTEN-FREE
CRACKERS OR USED AS A LOW-FAT SUBSTITUTE FOR MARGARINE OR BUTTER.

1 cup dried chickpeas
2 tbsp tahini GF
4 garlic cloves, crushed
4 tbsp lemon juice, plus extra (optional)
2 tbsp olive oil
2 tsp ground cumin
large pinch of cayenne pepper
½ tsp salt
paprika, to sprinkle
1 tbsp chopped parsley

PREP TIME: 20 MINUTES +
OVERNIGHT SOAKING
COOKING TIME: 1 ¼ HOURS
SERVINGS: 4

Put the chickpeas in a large bowl, cover with plenty of water and leave to soak overnight.
Drain, then rinse well.

Transfer the chickpeas to a large saucepan and cover with cold water. Bring to a boil, then
reduce the heat and simmer for 1 ¼ hours, or until the chickpeas are very tender, occasionally
skimming any froth from the surface. Drain well, reserving about 1 cup of the cooking liquid.
Leave the chickpeas until cool enough to handle. Pick over for any loose skins and discard.

Process the chickpeas, tahini, garlic, lemon juice, olive oil, cumin, salt and cayenne pepper in
a food processor until thick and smooth.With the motor still running, gradually add about ¾
cup of the reserved cooking liquid to form a smooth creamy purée. Add extra lemon juice, to
taste, if necessary.

Spread onto a flat bowl or plate, sprinkle with paprika and scatter the parsley over the top.

HINTS:
- Tahini is a thick paste made of ground sesame seeds. It is available at large supermarkets
  and health-food shops.
- Serve with vegetable crudités or gluten-free crackers.

nutrition per serving: Energy 58 Cal; Fat 3.7 g; Saturated fat 0.5 g; Protein 2.2 g; Carbohydrate 3.8 g;
Fiber 1.7 g; Cholesterol 0 mg

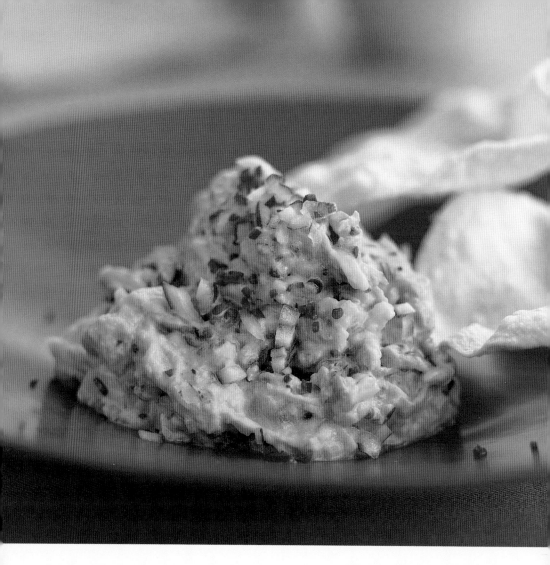

THIS LOW-FAT EGGPLANT
SAMBAL CAN BE SERVED AS A
SIDE DISH WITH CURRY AND
RICE OR ENJOYED AS A TASTY
DIP WITH GLUTEN-FREE BREAD,
CRACKERS OR POPPADOMS.

nutrition per serving: Energy 55 Cal

Fat 1.9 g

Saturated fat 0.6 g

Protein 3 g

Carbohydrate 5.9 g

Fiber 3.3 g

Cholesterol 4 mg

EGGPLANT SAMBAL

2 eggplants, halved
canola or olive oil spray
½ tsp ground turmeric
3 tbsp lime juice
2 red chilies, seeded and finely chopped
1 red onion, finely chopped
4 tbsp plain yogurt

PREP TIME: 15 MINUTES
COOKING TIME: 30 MINUTES
SERVINGS: 4

Preheat the oven to 400°F. Put the eggplants in a roasting pan, cut side up. Spray the cut halves of the eggplants with the oil and sprinkle with the turmeric. Roast for 30 minutes, or until they are browned all over and very soft.

Scoop the eggplant pulp into a bowl, then mash with the lime juice, chili and red onion, reserving some chili and onion for garnish.

Season with salt, then fold in the yogurt. Garnish with the remaining onion and chili.

HINTS:
- This is quite a chunky dip so it needs something crispy to scoop it up. Try gluten-free poppadoms or crackers.
- This dip can also be served as an accompaniment to curries or stir-fries, with some rice to provide a respite from the chili.

WHITE BEAN AND CHICKPEA DIP

THIS LOW-GI DIP IS A DELICIOUS WAY TO EAT LEGUMES. IT CAN BE SERVED
WITH FRESH VEGETABLES AND TOASTED GLUTEN-FREE TORTILLA PIECES AS A
SNACK OR USED IN PLACE OF MARGARINE OR BUTTER.

**15 oz canned cannellini (white) beans,
drained and rinsed**

15 oz canned chickpeas GF**, drained and
rinsed**

1½ tsp ground cumin

3 garlic cloves, crushed

2 tbsp chopped flat-leaf (Italian) parsley

3 tbsp lemon juice

1 tsp grated lemon zest

1 tbsp tahini GF

PREP TIME: 10 MINUTES
COOKING TIME: NONE
SERVINGS: 3—4

Place all ingredients in a food processor and process for 30 seconds. With the motor still running, slowly add 3 tablespoons hot water to the processor in a thin stream until the mixture is smooth and "dippable." Serve at room temperature with fresh vegetable sticks and gluten-free bread, crackers, rice cakes or toasted pieces of tortilla.

HINTS:
- Tahini is a thick paste made of ground sesame seeds. It is available at large supermarkets and health-food shops.
- Remember to read the ingredient list on the cans of cannellini beans and chickpeas to ensure that they are free of gluten; plain canned legumes usually are, but it's important to check in case a manufacturer uses a gluten-containing additive or preservative.

nutrition per serving: (4): Energy 167 Cal; Fat 4.7 g; Saturated fat 0.6 g; Protein 10.2 g; Carbohydrate 17.7 g; Fiber 8.3 g; Cholesterol 0 mg

MUSHROOM PÂTÉ

COMMERCIALLY MADE PÂTÉS CAN CONTAIN GLUTEN BUT YOU DON'T HAVE TO MISS OUT IF YOU MAKE YOUR OWN. THIS ONE IS SUITABLE FOR VEGETARIANS AND LOWER IN FAT THAN MANY COMMERCIAL VARIETIES.

1 tsp olive oil
1 small onion, chopped
2 garlic cloves, crushed
10½ oz flat mushrooms, wiped
   clean and chopped
4 tbsp dry white wine or water
1 cup fresh gluten-free breadcrumbs
2 tbsp thyme, plus extra to serve
2 tbsp chopped flat-leaf (Italian) parsley
1 tbsp lemon juice

PREP TIME: 15 MINUTES +
  1 HOUR REFRIGERATION
COOKING TIME: 10 MINUTES
SERVINGS: 4—6

Heat the oil in a large, deep frying pan. Add the onion and garlic and cook, stirring, for 2 minutes without browning. Add the mushrooms and white wine or water. Cook, stirring for 1 minute, then cover and simmer for 5 minutes, stirring once or twice. Remove the lid and increase the heat to evaporate any liquid. Cool.

Place the mushroom mixture, breadcrumbs, herbs and lemon juice in a food processor. Process until smooth and season well with salt and black pepper. Spoon into a serving bowl. Cover and refrigerate for at least 1 hour to allow the flavors to develop.

HINTS:
- You'll need about 3 average slices of gluten-free bread without crusts for the amount of breadcrumbs you need for the pâté. To make the breadcrumbs, blend the bread in a food processor until crumbs form.
- Serve with gluten-free bread or crackers.

nutrition per serving: (6): Energy 76 Cal; Fat 1.1 g; Saturated fat 0.2 g; Protein 3.3 g; Carbohydrate 10.1 g; Fiber 2.2 g; Cholesterol 1 mg

MINI POTATO AND LEEK QUICHES

3 to 4 boiling potatoes, peeled and chopped
2 tbsp canola or olive oil
2 cups gluten-free self-rising flour
1 tsp gluten-free baking powder
1 tsp salt
2 eggs

FILLING
3 tbsp butter
1 leek, washed and thinly sliced
3 eggs
¾ cup milk
¾ cup sour cream

PREP TIME: 20 MINUTES
COOKING TIME: 50 MINUTES
MAKES 24

Preheat the oven to 350°F. Lightly grease two 12-cup tart or muffin pans. Boil or steam the potatoes for 15 minutes, or until tender. Drain well, then mash until smooth. You will need 2 cups warm mashed potato for this recipe.

Combine the mashed potato and oil in a large bowl. Sift in the flour and baking powder, then add the salt and enough egg to mix to a smooth dough. Lightly dust a board with gluten-free flour, then knead the dough on this board until smooth. Roll out the pastry until it is ¼ in thick. Cut into 2½–2¾ in rounds and place in the prepared pans. Bake for 5 minutes, then remove from the oven and press out any air bubbles in the pastry. Cool completely. Increase the oven temperature to 400°F.

To make the filling, melt the butter in a heavy-based saucepan over medium heat. Add the leek and cook, stirring often, for 5–6 minutes until tender. Set aside to cool. Season with salt and freshly ground black pepper.

Whisk the eggs, milk and sour cream together in a bowl until well combined. Divide the leek mixture evenly among the pastry cases, then pour the egg mixture over the filling. Bake for 15–20 minutes, or until set and golden brown. Serve hot or cold.

HINTS:
- The quiches can be made the day before and refrigerated in an airtight container. Reheat for 10 minutes in a 300°F oven.
- These mini vegetarian quiches can be enjoyed as a light meal or served as finger food at a party. Enjoy in moderation because they are high in fat. You can use low-fat milk and light sour cream to lower the fat content if you are concerned about the fat content.

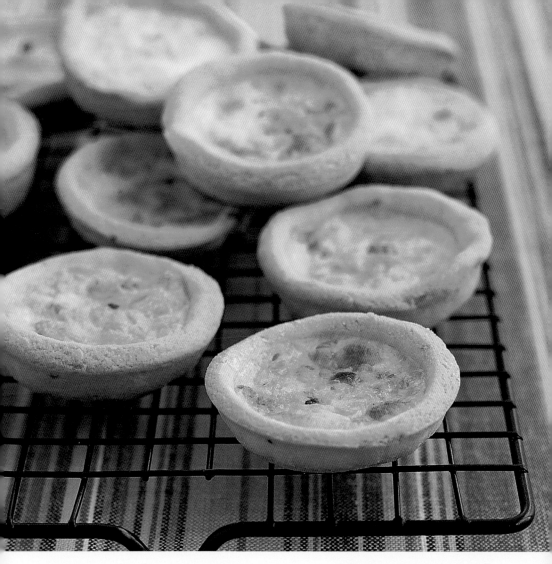

AFTER STARTING A GLUTEN-FREE
DIET YOU MAY HAVE THOUGHT
YOU'D NEVER BE ABLE TO ENJOY
QUICHE AGAIN, BUT IT'S EASY TO
MAKE A GLUTEN-FREE VERSION.

nutrition per quiche: Energy 138 Cal

Fat 7.7 g

Saturated fat 3.7 g

Protein 3 g

Carbohydrate 13.7 g

Fiber 1.5 g

Cholesterol 55 mg

MINI SWEET POTATO QUICHES

THESE MINI QUICHES CAN BE SERVED AS A SNACK OR FINGER FOOD, BUT DON'T GO OVERBOARD BECAUSE THEY'RE NOT LOW IN CALORIES. YOU CAN USE LOW-FAT MILK AND LIGHT SOUR CREAM TO LOWER THE FAT CONTENT.

3 cups gluten-free all-purpose flour
¾ cup + 2 tbsp butter
2 eggs, lightly beaten

SWEET POTATO FILLING
1 large sweet potato, peeled and cut into ½ in dice
canola or olive oil spray

7 oz ricotta cheese, crumbled
2 tbsp snipped chives
3 eggs
¾ cup milk
¾ cup sour cream

PREP TIME: 25 MINUTES
COOKING TIME: 35 MINUTES
MAKES 24

Preheat the oven to 400°F. Lightly grease a baking tray and two 12-cup muffin or tart pans.

Sift the flour into a large bowl. Rub in the butter with your fingertips until the mixture resembles dry breadcrumbs. Make a well in the center and add the lightly beaten eggs and 1–2 tablespoons water, or enough to form a soft dough. Lightly dust a board with gluten-free flour, then put the dough on the board and knead lightly. Lightly dust two large sheets of baking paper with gluten-free flour, then roll out the pastry between these sheets to about ⅛ in thick. Cut the dough into 2½–2¾ in rounds and place in the prepared patty pans. The dough should make 24 rounds.

To make the sweet potato filling, put the sweet potato on the prepared tray. Spray with oil and season with a little salt and pepper. Bake for 15 minutes, or until golden brown. Cool. Combine the sweet potato with the crumbled ricotta cheese and snipped chives.

Combine the eggs, milk and sour cream in a bowl until well combined. Divide the sweet potato mixture evenly among the pastry cases, then pour the egg mixture over the filling. Bake for 15–20 minutes, or until golden brown. Serve hot or cold.

HINT:
• The quiches can be made the day before and refrigerated in an airtight container. Reheat for 10 minutes in a 300°F oven.

nutrition per quiche: Energy 205 Cal; Fat 12.7 g; Saturated fat 7.7 g; Protein 3.2 g; Carbohydrate 19.3 g; Fiber 0.6 g; Cholesterol 76 mg.

CRISPY WAFER COOKIES

THESE LIGHT CRISPY COOKIES ARE GOOD ON THEIR OWN OR SERVED WITH ONE OF THE DIPS ON THE PREVIOUS PAGES. IF YOU HAVE KIDS WHO NEED GLUTEN-FREE SNACKS YOU'LL BE ASKED TO MAKE THESE REGULARLY.

1 cup rice flour
1 cup pure maize cornstarch GF
½ cup rice bran
½ tsp salt
2 tbsp canola or olive oil

PREP TIME: 10 MINUTES
COOKING TIME: 25 MINUTES
MAKES ABOUT 40

Preheat the oven to 400°F. Lightly grease two 9 x 13 in pans.

Combine the dry ingredients in a bowl and make a well in the middle. In a separate bowl mix together ¾ cup water and the oil, then pour into the well in the dry ingredients. Mix until thoroughly combined.

Divide the mixture into two portions. Press each portion of dough into one of the prepared pans and bake for 20–25 minutes. Cool in the pan. Break into pieces and store in an airtight container for up to 2 days.

HINT:
• If you'd like more evenly shaped cookies, score the dough in the tins with a knife before you bake them, then the cookies will be easy to break neatly once they're cooked.

nutrition per serving: Energy 41 Cal; Fat 1.3 g; Saturated fat 0.2 g; Protein 0.4 g; Carbohydrate 6.6 g; Fiber 0.4 g; Cholesterol 0 mg

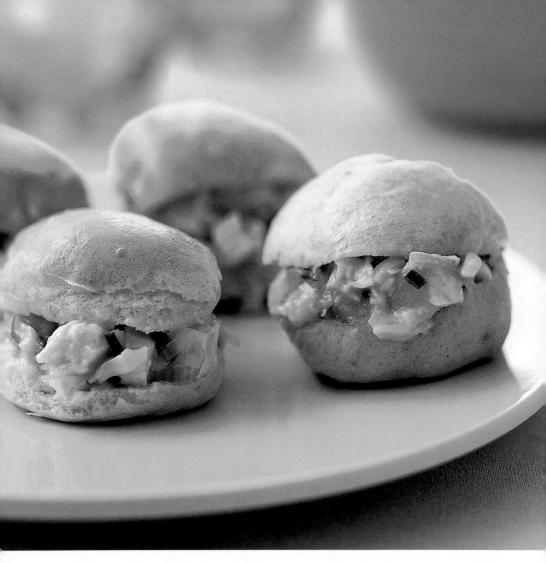

THESE WILL BE HARD TO RESIST
WHETHER YOU NEED A GLUTENFREE
DIET OR NOT. TAKE A PLATE OF
THESE WITH YOU WHEN YOU'RE
INVITED TO A FRIEND'S HOUSE, SO
THERE'S SOMETHING SUITABLE FOR
YOU TO EAT—BUT BE PREPARED TO
FIGHT FOR THEM.

nutrition per serving: Energy 78 Cal
Fat 5.3 g
Saturated fat 1.5 g
Protein 2.6 g
Carbohydrate 5 g
Fiber 0.2 g
Cholesterol 32 mg

CHICKEN AND LEEK PUFFS

4 tbsp canola or olive oil
¾ cup gluten-free all-purpose flour
¼ tsp baking soda
¾ tsp gluten-free baking powder
3 eggs

CHICKEN AND LEEK FILLING
3 tbsp butter
6 boneless, skinless chicken breast
½ leek, washed and thinly sliced
1 tbsp gluten-free all-purpose flour

3 tbsp milk
3 tbsp chicken stock GF (Basics)
1 tbsp chopped parsley

PREP TIME: 1 HOUR
COOKING TIME: 40 MINUTES
MAKES 24

Preheat the oven to 415°F. Cover two baking trays with baking paper. Pour 1 cup water and the oil into a saucepan and bring to a boil. Remove from the heat, add the sifted dry ingredients, then return to the heat and stir constantly until the mixture thickens and leaves the side of the saucepan (it may look a little oily). Scoop into the small bowl of an electric mixer and set aside to cool slightly.

Beat the mixture, adding the eggs one at a time and beating well between each addition, until it is thick and shiny. Place level tablespoons of the mixture onto the prepared trays. Spray lightly all over with cold water, to aid rising. Bake for 10 minutes, or until they rise and start to brown. Reduce the heat to 375°F and bake for 10–15 minutes, or until cooked through. Remove the puffs from the oven and leave to cool on a wire rack.

To make the chicken and leek filling, melt 1 tablespoon of the butter in a frying pan over medium heat, add the chicken breast and fry for 3 minutes on each side, or until cooked through. Remove from the pan and cut into small pieces. Melt the remaining butter in a saucepan, add the leek and cook, stirring often, for 5–6 minutes, or until soft. Sprinkle the flour over the leek and cook, stirring, for 20 seconds. Add the combined milk and stock, stirring over the heat until the mixture boils and thickens. Season with a little salt and pepper. Add the chicken and parsley to the sauce and heat gently until warmed through.

Split the puffs in half, spoon in the warm filling, then replace the tops. Serve while warm.

HINT:
• The puffs can be made and stored unfilled in an airtight container for 1 week. If they become soft, reheat them in a 300°F oven for 5–10 minutes.

GLAZED DRUMSTICKS

THESE DRUMSTICKS WILL SUIT PEOPLE WHO ALSO HAVE OTHER FOOD INTOLERANCES BECAUSE THEY ARE FREE OF WHEAT, GLUTEN, NUT, EGG AND DAIRY. THEY ARE A GOOD ADDITION TO A LUNCH BOX OR PICNIC HAMPER.

8 large chicken drumsticks (skin removed)
4 tbsp golden syrup or honey
3 tbsp pear juice
1 tbsp canola or olive oil
1 tsp salt

PREP TIME: 20 MINUTES +
  OVERNIGHT MARINATING
COOKING TIME: 40 MINUTES
SERVINGS: 4

Put the drumsticks in a shallow non-metallic dish. Combine the remaining ingredients and pour the marinade over the drumsticks, making sure they are all coated. Marinate overnight, turning occasionally.

Preheat the oven to 350°F. Put the drumsticks and marinade into a baking dish. Bake for 35–40 minutes, turning frequently during cooking and brushing with the pan juices. If the pan juices start to overbrown, add a small amount of water or stock until syrupy. Serve hot or cold.

HINT:
• Serve these as a snack or with a selection of salads for a meal.

nutrition per serving: Energy 552 Cal; Fat 23.5 g; Saturated fat 5.8 g; Protein 62.4 g; Carbohydrate 23.8 g; Fiber 0 g; Cholesterol 267 mg

VEAL AND CHICKEN TERRINE

COMMERCIAL TERRINES AND PÂTÉS MAY CONTAIN GLUTEN. MAKE YOUR OWN
TO ENSURE YOU'RE GETTING A GLUTEN-FREE VERSION

2 tbsp canola or olive oil

2 garlic cloves, crushed

1 leek, washed and finely chopped

about 2 lbs minced (ground) veal

1 handful snipped chives

3 eggs, lightly beaten

2 tbsp canola or olive oil, extra

3 tbsp gin

1½ tsp salt

½ cup fresh gluten-free breadcrumbs

2 boneless, skinless chicken breasts, each
   cut into four long strips

PREP TIME: 45 MINUTES
COOKING TIME: 1 ½ HOURS
SERVINGS: 6–8

Preheat the oven to 350°F. Grease a 8 x 4 in loaf pan, then line with foil.

Heat the oil in a frying pan over medium heat, add the garlic and leek and fry for about
5 minutes, or until soft. Allow to cool. Transfer to a bowl, then add the veal, chives, eggs,
extra oil, gin, salt and breadcrumbs. Using your hands, mix and knead the mixture until it is
well combined.

Put half of the mince mixture into the prepared pan, pressing down well. Lay the chicken
breast strips over the meat. Press the remaining mince mixture over the chicken. Cover with
greased foil. Place in a baking dish and add enough boiling water to come halfway up the
sides of the loaf pan. Bake for 1¼–1½ hours.

When cooked, remove the loaf pan from the dish of water and drain off any liquid. Put
a piece of cardboard on top of the terrine, then weigh it down with a heavy weight (for
instance, cans of food). Refrigerate until cold.

HINTS:
- Make your own breadcrumbs by blending gluten-free bread in a food processor until
  crumbs form.you'fll need about 1½ pieces of gluten-free bread without crusts to make
  enough for this recipe.
- Cut into thin slices and serve with salad or use as a sandwich filling.

nutrition per serving: (8): Energy 382 Cal; Fat 20.6 g; Saturated fat 5.2 g; Protein 41.1 g;
Carbohydrate 4.3 g; Fiber 0.5 g; Cholesterol 205 mg

ROAST PUMPKIN AND FETA PIZZA

3 cups gluten-free all-purpose flour

4 tsp dried yeast ^{GF}

½ tsp sugar

1 tsp salt

1½ tbsp canola or olive oil

TOPPING

about 1 lb pumpkin or winter squash,
   peeled, seeded and chopped

canola or olive oil spray

1 tbsp canola or olive oil

2 onions, thinly sliced

2 garlic cloves, crushed

3 tbsp pine nuts

3 tbsp tomato paste ^{GF}

1 garlic clove, extra, crushed

1 tsp dried oregano

4½ oz reduced-fat feta cheese, crumbled

4 tbsp black olives, pitted and crushed

2 tbsp thyme

PREP TIME: 45 MINUTES +
   1 HOUR RISING

COOKING TIME: 1 HOUR 5 MINUTES

SERVINGS: 4

Combine the yeast, sugar and 3 tablespoons warm water in a small bowl and set aside until foaming. Sift the flour and salt into a large bowl. In a separate bowl mix together 1 cup warm water and the oil, then pour into the well in the dry ingredients along with the yeast mixture. Use a wooden spoon to mix until almost combined. Use your hands to mix into a soft dough.

Lightly dust a board with gluten-free flour. Turn the dough out onto the board and knead until smooth. Place the dough in a lightly oiled bowl. Cover and set aside in a warm place for 1 hour, or until the dough has doubled in size.

Meanwhile, make the topping. Preheat the oven to 350°F. Line a baking tray with baking paper. Put the pumpkin on the lined tray and spray with oil. Bake for 45 minutes. Set aside. Increase the oven temperature to 425°F. While the pumpkin is cooking, heat the oil in a large non-stick frying pan over medium heat. Add the onion and garlic and cook, stirring often, for 5 minutes, or until the onion is very soft. Stir in the pine nuts, remove from the heat and set aside. In a small bowl combine the tomato paste, garlic and oregano with 1 tablespoon water.

Use your fist to punch the dough down, then knead until it returns to its original size. Lightly grease two 10¾ in pizza trays. Divide the dough into two portions. On a surface lightly dusted with gluten-free flour, roll out one portion to fit the tray, then carefully place the dough onto the tray. Repeat with the remaining dough. Spread the tomato paste mixture evenly over each pizza base, then spread the onion mixture over this. Scatter the pumpkin, feta, olives and thyme over the top. Bake for 20 minutes, swapping the trays around once, or until the dough is golden.

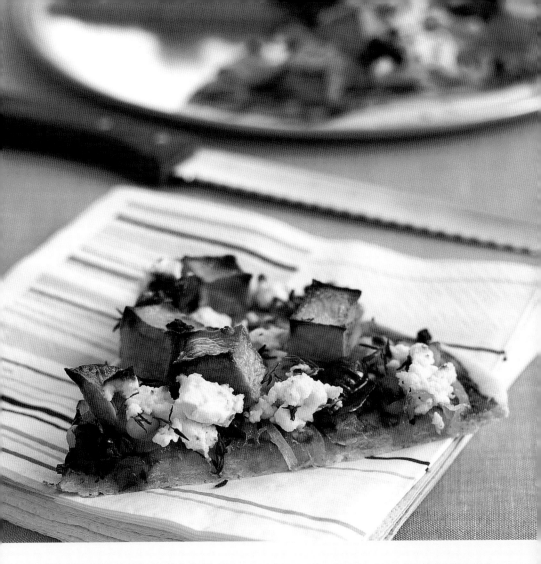

HERE'S A RECIPE FOR A GLUTENFREE
GOURMET PIZZA THAT IS A GREAT
SOURCE OF THE ANTIOXIDANT
BETACAROTENE, THANKS TO THE
PUMPKIN. EXPERIMENT WITH
DIFFERENT FLOURS TO FIND THE
BEST ONE.

nutrition per serving: Energy 815 Cal

Fat 30.3 g

Saturated fat 7.6 g

Protein 13.9 g

Carbohydrate 117.2 g

Fiber 6.4 g

Cholesterol 22 mg

RICE AND COTTAGE CHEESE PIE

RICE IS AN IMPORTANT FOOD FOR PEOPLE ON GLUTEN-FREE DIETS AND CAN BE PREPARED IN MANY DIFFERENT WAYS. IN THIS RECIPE, RICE FORMS THE BASE OF A DELICIOUS PIE THAT CAN BE EATEN WARM OR COLD.

½ cup white long-grain rice

2 tbsp snipped chives

2 tbsp butter, melted

4 tbsp cottage cheese

2 eggs, lightly beaten

PREP TIME: 40 MINUTES + COOLING
COOKING TIME: 1 HOUR
SERVINGS: 4—6

FILLING

4 tbsp butter

5 spring onions (scallions), sliced

4 eggs

1 cup cottage cheese

Preheat the oven to 325°F. Lightly grease a 9 in pie plate.

Bring a large saucepan of water to the boil. Add the rice and cook for 12 minutes, or until very tender, stirring occasionally. Drain and cool. You will need 1½ cups of cold cooked rice for this recipe. Combine the cooled rice with the chives, butter, cottage cheese and eggs and press into the base and sides of the prepared tin. Chill for 30 minutes.

Meanwhile, prepare the filling. Melt the butter in a small saucepan over low heat. Add the spring onion and cook for 8–10 minutes, or until soft, but not brown. Remove from the heat. Allow to cool.

Combine the eggs, cottage cheese and a pinch of salt in a bowl. Add the spring onion mixture and mix well. Pour the filling into the prepared crust. Bake for 40–45 minutes, or until firm and golden brown. Serve hot or cold.

HINTS:

• The rice should be very well cooked and slightly mushy. This can be achieved by stirring it once or twice during cooking.

• If you have diabetes, use a lower GI rice, such as basmati, koshikari or doongara.

• Serve the pie with a salad or on its own.

nutrition per serving: (6): Energy 307 Cal; Fat 20.4 g; Saturated fat 11.6 g; Protein 15.7 g; Carbohydrate 15 g; Fiber 0.5 g; Cholesterol 240 mg

SPICY LENTIL SALAD

LENTILS, LIKE ALL LEGUMES, ARE A NATURAL SUPER FOOD—THEY'RE LOW GI, A GREAT SOURCE OF FIBER, AND PROVIDE GOOD AMOUNTS OF VITAMINS, MINERALS AND ANTIOXIDANTS.

1 heaping cup basmati rice
1 cup brown lentils
1 tsp ground turmeric
1 tsp ground cinnamon
6 cardamom pods
3 star anise
2 bay leaves
3 tbsp canola or olive oil
1 tbsp lemon juice
1 cup broccoli florets
2 carrots, peeled and cut into
    julienne strips
1 onion, finely chopped
2 garlic cloves, crushed
1 red pepper, finely chopped

1 tsp garam masala
1 tsp ground coriander
1⅔ cups fresh or frozen peas, thawed if
    frozen

DRESSING
1 cup plain yogurt
1 tbsp lemon juice
1 tbsp chopped mint
1 tsp cumin seeds

PREP TIME: 30 MINUTES
COOKING TIME: 1 ¼ HOURS
SERVINGS: 6

Put the rice, lentils, turmeric, cinnamon, cardamom pods, star anise and bay leaves in a saucepan with 3 cups water. Stir well and bring to a boil. Reduce the heat, cover and simmer gently for 50–60 minutes, or until the liquid is absorbed. Remove the whole spices. Transfer the mixture to a large bowl. Whisk 2 tablespoons of the oil with the lemon juice, then fork through the rice mixture.

Steam or boil the broccoli and carrots until tender. Drain and refresh in cold water.

Heat the remaining oil in a large frying pan and add the onion, garlic and pepper. Stir-fry for 2–3 minutes, then add the garam masala and coriander and stir-fry for a further 1–2 minutes. Add the cooked vegetables and peas and toss to coat in the spice mixture. Add to the rice and fork through to combine. Cover and refrigerate until cold.

To make the dressing, mix the yogurt, lemon juice, mint and cumin seeds together, then season with salt and freshly ground black pepper. Spoon the salad into six individual bowls or onto a platter and top with the dressing.

nutrition per serving: Energy 381 Cal; Fat 12 g; Saturated fat 1.4 g; Protein 17.4 g; Carbohydrate 51.5 g; Fiber 11.2 g; Cholesterol 4 mg

71

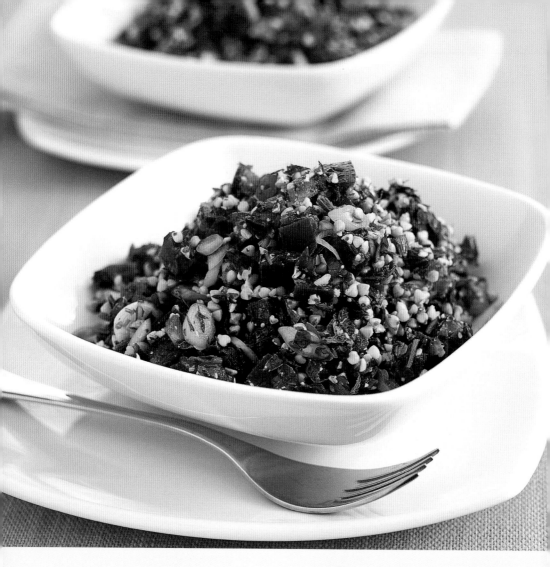

IF YOU'RE NEW TO GLUTEN-FREE
COOKING AND STILL WONDERING
HOW YOU CAN USE INGREDIENTS
LIKE BUCKWHEAT, TRY THIS RECIPE.
IT'S A GLUTEN-FREE VERSION OF
TABOULEH. IT'S VERY VERSATILE
AND CAN BE EATEN AS A SNACK,
SANDWICH FILLING OR SIDE SALAD.

nutrition per serving (6): Energy 179 Cal
Fat 7.1 g
Saturated fat 1 g
Protein 5.2 g
Carbohydrate 20.9 g
Fiber 5.8 g
Cholesterol 0 mg

ROASTED BUCKWHEAT TABOULEH

1 cup roasted buckwheat kernels (groats)
2 large bunches flat-leaf (Italian) parsley
1 handful mint
4 spring onions (scallions), thinly sliced
4 tomatoes, finely chopped
2 garlic cloves, crushed
3 tbsp lemon juice
2 tbsp olive oil

PREP TIME: 30 MINUTES +
15 MINUTES SOAKING
COOKING TIME: NONE
SERVINGS: 4–6

Put the buckwheat in a bowl. Pour in enough water to cover the buckwheat and leave to soak for 15 minutes, or until the buckwheat has softened a little. Drain well, then spread onto a clean dish towel to dry.

Finely chop the parsley and mint with a large knife or in a food processor. If you are using a food processor, take care not to over-process.

Put the buckwheat, herbs, spring onion and tomato in a large bowl. To make the dressing, combine the garlic, lemon juice and oil in a jar with a tight-fitting lid and shake well. Pour the dressing over the salad and toss well. Refrigerate until required. Return to room temperature to serve.

HINTS:
- Buckwheat kernels are the inner shell of the husked buckwheat grain—the outer husk is inedible. Roasted buckwheat kernels look like little stones and can be bought from health-food stores. Raw buckwheat kernels can taste slightly bitter so if you buy unroasted buckwheat kernels, dry-roast them for a few minutes. It may take you a little while to get used to the crunch of the buckwheat.
- If you like, you can boost the flavor of the salad by using 3 garlic cloves, doubling the amount of lemon juice and adding an extra tablespoon of olive oil

CANNELLINI BEAN AND ARUGULA SALAD

THIS COLORFUL SALAD CAN BE SERVED AS A SIDE DISH, SNACK OR LIGHT
VEGETARIAN MEAL.

3 red peppers, halved and seeded
1 garlic clove, crushed
grated zest of 1 lemon
2 handfuls coarsely chopped flat-leaf
(Italian) parsley
15 oz canned cannellini (white)
beans ^{GF}, drained and rinsed
2 tbsp lemon juice
2 tbsp extra-virgin olive oil

1 small bunch arugula or mixed salad
leaves

PREP TIME: 20 MINUTES
COOKING TIME: 15 MINUTES
SERVINGS: 2 AS AMAIN COURSE OR
4 AS A STARTER

Preheat a grill or broiler to medium. Roast the peppers, skin side up, until the skin blackens and blisters. Set aside in a plastic bag for 5 minutes, then peel away the skin and slice the flesh into strips.

Combine the garlic, lemon zest and parsley in a bowl.

Put the cannellini beans in a bowl and add half of the parsley mixture, 1 tablespoon lemon juice, 1 tablespoon extra-virgin olive oil and salt and pepper to taste. Toss together. Place the salad leaves on a large plate and dress with the remaining lemon juice and extra-virgin olive oil.

Scatter the bean mixture over the leaves, then lay the pepper strips on top, along with the remaining parsley mixture. Season with salt and pepper and serve immediately.

HINTS:
• When using canned beans, check the label to ensure that the manufacturer has not used any additives that contain gluten.
• Instead of canned beans, you can soak 1 ¼ cups dried beans overnight, then boil with a dash of oil and no salt for 30–40 minutes, or until tender.
• The red peppers, herbs and lemon juice add vitamin C, which can help the amount of iron you absorb from the beans.

nutrition per serving (4): Energy 174 Cal; Fat 9.7 g; Saturated fat 1.3 g; Protein 7.1 g; Carbohydrate 12.4 g; Fiber 5.9 g; Cholesterol 0 mg

ROAST MUSHROOM AND BABY BEAN SALAD

THIS SALAD IS A GOOD SOURCE OF B-GROUP VITAMINS, MAKING IT A WISE CHOICE FOR PEOPLE RECOVERING FROM LONG-STANDING CELIAC DISEASE.

1 lb 5 oz field mushrooms, brushed clean

2 tbsp olive oil

3 garlic cloves, crushed

2 tbsp lemon juice

6 French shallots, root ends trimmed, skin left on

1½ tbsp tarragon vinegar

2 tsp finely chopped tarragon

1 tbsp finely chopped flat-leaf (Italian) parsley

1 cup baby green beans, trimmed

2 handfuls arugula

PREP TIME: 15 MINUTES

COOKING TIME: 35 MINUTES

SERVINGS: 4

Preheat the oven to 400°F. Place the mushrooms in a single layer in a large roasting pan. Add the oil, garlic, lemon juice and shallots and gently toss until coated. Roast for 30 minutes, occasionally spooning over the juices. Remove from the oven and cool to room temperature. Slip the shallots from their skins and discard the skin.

Pour the cooking juices into a large mixing bowl. Add the tarragon vinegar, tarragon and parsley. Mix and season well.

Blanch the beans in boiling salted water for 2 minutes, or until just tender. Drain well and, while still hot, add to the dressing. Set aside to cool to room temperature.

Cut the mushrooms into quarters, or eighths if large, and add to the beans along with the shallots and arugula. Gently toss together and serve on a platter or four individual plates.

HINT:
- Tarragon vinegar is available at most supermarkets or delicatessens. Alternatively, use white wine vinegar if tarragon vinegar is not available. Do not use malt vinegar because it contains gluten.

nutrition per serving: Energy 151 Cal; Fat 9.9 g; Saturated fat 1.3 g; Protein 7.3 g; Carbohydrate 4.8 g; Fiber 6.2 g; Cholesterol 0 mg

POTATO AND PUMPKIN SOUP

1 tbsp canola or olive oil
1 leek, halved lengthways, washed
   and sliced
2 garlic cloves, crushed
2 potatoes, peeled and chopped
1 large butternut squash, peeled, seeded
   and chopped
5 cups vegetable stock ^{GF} (Basics)
snipped chives, to serve
gluten-free bread, to serve

PREP TIME: 30 MINUTES
COOKING TIME: 40 MINUTES
SERVINGS: 4

Heat the oil in a large saucepan over medium heat. Add the leek and garlic and cook, stirring, for 2 minutes. Reduce the heat to low. Cover the pan with a lid and cook, stirring occasionally, for 7–8 minutes, or until the leek is very soft.

Add the potato, pumpkin and stock to the pan. Bring to a boil. Reduce the heat and simmer, partially covered, for 20–25 minutes, or until the vegetables are very soft. Set the pan aside for 10 minutes to allow the mixture to cool slightly.

Purée the soup in a blender or food processor (in batches, if necessary) until smooth. Divide the soup among four bowls and sprinkle with chives. Serve with gluten-free bread.

HINTS:

- If you're using a commercial stock, check the label to ensure it has no ingredients that contain gluten. Even better, make your own—it is much healthier and you can ensure that it contains no gluten.
- If you can tolerate dairy foods, add 2 teaspoons of light sour cream or plain yogurt to each bowl of soup before serving.
- Diabetics should limit their intake of this soup because it has a relatively high-GI value (due to the potatoes and pumpkin) so will cause a high blood-sugar response.

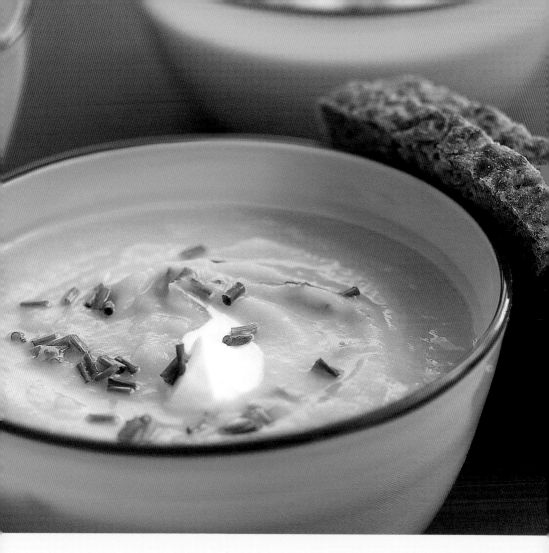

This vibrant soup can be served as a starter, snack or meal (add some gluten-free bread). It may be particularly appealing to fussy eaters as it's a relatively simple soup.

nutrition per serving: Energy 200 Cal
Fat 6.2 g
Saturated fat 1.1 g
Protein 6.2 g
Carbohydrate 27.7 g
Fiber 7 g
Cholesterol 25 mg

FISH AND BEAN SOUP

MANY PEOPLE DON'T EAT THE THREE OR MORE SERVES OF FISH EACH WEEK THAT IS RECOMMENDED BY NUTRITIONISTS. THIS SOUP IS A DELICIOUS AND SIMPLE WAY FOR YOU TO INCLUDE FISH IN YOUR DIET.

2 tbsp canola or olive oil

1 large leek, washed and thinly sliced

2–3 boiling potatoes, peeled and chopped

2 garlic cloves, crushed

6 cups chicken stock GF (Basics)

1 cup green beans, cut into 1¼ in pieces

**about 1 lb firm white boneless fish,
    cut into small cubes**

**3 spring onions (scallions), thinly sliced
    diagonally**

PREP TIME: 15 MINUTES
COOKING TIME: 30 MINUTES
SERVINGS: 4

Heat the oil in a large saucepan over medium heat. Cook the leek, stirring often, for 5–6 minutes, or until it softens.

Add the potato and garlic and cook, stirring, for 2 minutes. Pour in the stock, increase the heat to high and bring to a boil. Reduce the heat and simmer, partially covered, for 10 minutes, or until the potato is almost tender when tested with the point of a knife.

Add the beans and fish and continue to cook for a further 5 minutes, or until the fish and beans are cooked. Stir in the spring onions. Season to taste with salt and pepper.

HINTS:
- Many commercial stocks contain gluten. If you are not using homemade stock, check the ingredient list carefully.
- If you have diabetes, you can replace the high-GI potatoes with a lower GI alternative, such as canned chickpeas or cannellini (white) beans; this will ensure your blood-sugar response is not as high.

nutrition per serving: Energy 355 Cal; Fat 12.7 g; Saturated fat 2 g; Protein 36 g; Carbohydrate 21.8 g; Fiber 4.8 g; Cholesterol 81 mg

RED LENTIL AND PARSNIP SOUP

THIS HEARTY SOUP IS A GREAT WAY TO EAT SEVERAL DIFFERENT VEGETABLES IN ONE MEAL. IF YOU HAVE DIABETES, YOU CAN LOWER THE SOUP'S GI BY SWAPPING THE PARSNIP WITH A SMALL SWEET POTATO.

1 tsp olive oil
1 onion, chopped
2 garlic cloves, crushed
1 parsnip, peeled and chopped
1 celery stalk, chopped
1 large carrot, peeled and chopped
1 tsp ground cumin
1 tbsp tomato paste GF
14 oz canned diced tomatoes
¾ cup red lentils

4 cups chicken or vegetable stock GF
 (Basics) or water
1 tbsp lemon juice
1 handful chopped flat-leaf (Italian) parsley
gluten-free bread, to serve

PREP TIME: 20 MINUTES
COOKING TIME: 30 MINUTES
SERVINGS: 4

Heat the oil in a large, heavy-based saucepan. Add the onion and garlic and stir-fry for 2 minutes, or until softened. Add the parsnip, celery and carrot and cook, covered, over low heat for 8 minutes to sweat the vegetables. Stir once or twice, taking care not to brown.

Stir in the cumin, tomato paste, tomatoes, lentils and stock or water. Bring to a boil, then reduce the heat and simmer for 20 minutes, or until the lentils are cooked. Season well with salt and pepper. Stir in the lemon juice and parsley. Serve with gluten-free bread.

HINTS:
• If you're using a commercial brand of stock check the label to ensure it is free of gluten.
• This is a thick soup; if you prefer, add more stock or water to make it thinner.
• You can freeze the soup in serving-sized portions for up to 1 month.

nutrition per serving: 232 Cal; Fat 2.8 g; Saturated fat 0.4 g; Protein 17.3 g; Carbohydrate 30.5 g; Fiber 10 g; Cholesterol 5 mg

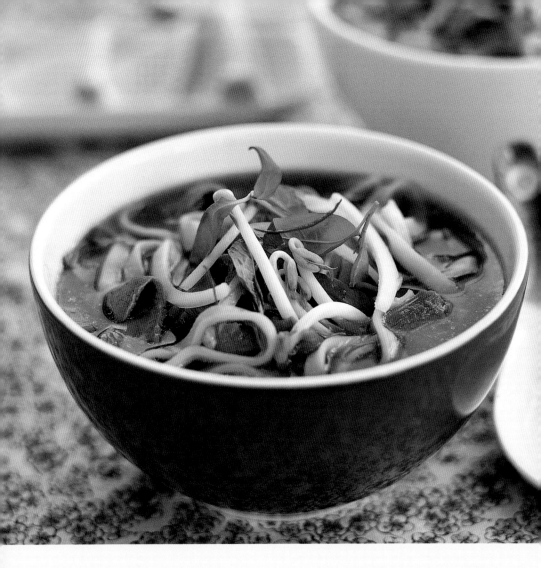

TAKE YOUR TASTE BUDS ON AN
EXOTIC JOURNEY WITH THIS CLASSIC
ASIAN SOUP. IT'S A COMPLETE LOW-
GI MEAL IN A BOWL THAT PROVIDES
GOOD AMOUNTS OF IRON, ZINC,
VITAMIN B12 AND FOLATE. THE
FRAGRANT HERBS AND SPICES WILL
AWAKEN YOUR SENSES.

nutrition per serving: Energy 326 Cal

Fat 6.1 g

Saturated fat 2.4 g

Protein 31.2 g

Carbohydrate 35.9 g

Fiber 2.5 g

Cholesterol 64 mg

VIETNAMESE BEEF SOUP

about 1 lb lean rump steak, trimmed
½ onion
1½ tbsp fish sauce GF
1 star anise
1 cinnamon stick
pinch of ground white pepper
6 cups beef stock GF **(Basics)**
10½ oz thin fresh rice noodles
3 spring onions (scallions), thinly sliced
1 small handful Vietnamese mint
1 cup bean sprouts, trimmed

1 small onion, halved and thinly sliced
1 small red chili, thinly sliced diagonally
lemon wedges, to serve

PREP TIME: 20 MINUTES +
   40 MINUTES FREEZING
COOKING TIME: 30 MINUTES
SERVINGS: 4

Wrap the steak in plastic wrap and freeze for 40 minutes. Freezing the meat will make it easier to slice.

Meanwhile, put the onion half, fish sauce, star anise, cinnamon stick, white pepper, stock and 2 cups water in a large saucepan. Bring to a boil, then reduce the heat, cover and simmer for 20 minutes. Discard the onion, star anise and cinnamon stick.

Put the noodles in a large heatproof bowl. Cover with boiling water and soak for 5 minutes, or until softened. Separate gently and drain. Thinly slice the meat across the grain.

Divide the noodles and spring onion among four deep bowls. Top with the beef, mint, bean sprouts, thinly sliced onion and chili. Ladle the hot broth over the top and serve with the lemon wedges—the heat of the liquid will cook the beef.

HINTS:
- Fish sauce can be a hidden source of gluten. When you dine out at an Asian restaurant, check that they use a gluten-free fish sauce.
- Some brands of stock (ready-to-use, cubes and powder) are not free of gluten, so check the ingredient list if you are using a commercial brand.
- Vietnamese mint has thin, pointed leaves and a strong peppery, minty flavor. If you can't find it, use regular mint instead.
- People with long-standing celiac disease often become iron deficient. This soup is a good way to add more iron-rich foods to your diet.

MAIN MEALS

SPICY VEGETABLE STEW WITH DAL

SERVE WITH BASMATI RICE FOR A BALANCED, LOW-GI VEGETARIAN MEAL. THE SPICES ADD COLOR AND FLAVOR AND USEFUL AMOUNTS OF MANY MINERALS. BOTH THE DAL AND STEW ARE DELICIOUS REHEATED THE NEXT DAY.

DAL
⅔ cup yellow split peas
2 in piece of fresh ginger, grated
2–3 garlic cloves, crushed
1 red chili, seeded and chopped

3 tomatoes
1 red onion
¼ cauliflower
3 slender eggplants
2 carrots, peeled
2 small zucchini
2 tsp canola or olive oil

1 tsp yellow mustard seeds
1 tsp cumin seeds
1 tsp ground cumin
½ tsp garam masala
1½ cups vegetable stock GF (Basics)
½ cup frozen peas, thawed
1 large handful cilantro leaves

PREP TIME: 25 MINUTES +
   2 HOURS SOAKING
COOKING TIME: 1 ½ HOURS
SERVINGS 4

To make the dal, put the split peas in a bowl, cover with water and soak for 2 hours. Drain. Put in a large saucepan with the ginger, garlic, chili and 3 cups water. Bring to a boil, then reduce the heat and simmer for 40 minutes, or until just soft.

Meanwhile, prepare the vegetables. To peel the tomatoes, score a cross in the base of each one. Cover with boiling water for 30 seconds, then plunge into cold water. Drain and peel away the skin from the cross. Scoop out the seeds with a teaspoon and roughly chop the flesh. Cut the onion into thin wedges, cut the cauliflower into florets and thickly slice the eggplants, carrots and zucchini.

Heat the oil in a large saucepan over medium heat. Add the mustard seeds, cumin seeds, ground cumin and garam masala and cook for 30 seconds, or until fragrant. Add the onion and cook for a further 2 minutes, or until the onion is soft. Stir in the tomato, eggplant, carrot and cauliflower.

Add the dal and stock, mix together well and simmer, covered, for 45 minutes, or until the vegetables are tender. Stir occasionally. Add the zucchini and peas during the last 10 minutes of cooking. Stir in the cilantro leaves and serve hot.

nutrition per serving: Energy 204 Cal; Fat 4.3 g; Saturated fat 0.5 g; Protein 14.1 g; Carbohydrate 27.8 g; Fiber 10 g; Cholesterol 0 mg

BEEF AND SPINACH LASAGNA

THIS GLUTEN-FREE VERSION OF LASAGNA CAN BE ENJOYED BY THE WHOLE FAMILY. THERE'S NO NEED TO COOK SEPARATE VERSIONS FOR THOSE WHO CAN EAT GLUTEN AND THOSE WHO CAN'T.

1 tbsp canola or olive oil

1 large onion, finely chopped

3 large garlic cloves, crushed

1 celery stalk, diced

about 1 lb lean minced (ground) beef

1 tsp dried oregano

28 oz canned diced tomatoes

2 tbsp tomato paste GF

1 cup) beef stock GF (Basics) or water

1 bunch English spinach, stalks removed, washed

16 oz gluten-free lasagna sheets

WHITE SAUCE

3 tbsp pure maize cornstarch GF

1½ cups reduced-fat milk

1 slice of onion

½ tsp ground nutmeg

⅔ cup ricotta cheese

¾ cup firmly packed grated cheddar cheese GF

PREP TIME: 30 MINUTES

COOKING TIME: 1 ¾ HOURS

SERVINGS 6—8

Heat the oil in a large, non-stick saucepan. Add the onion and cook for 2 minutes. Add the garlic and celery and cook for a further 2 minutes. Add the beef and oregano and cook over high heat for 5 minutes, or until cooked, breaking up any lumps with a spoon. Add the tomatoes, tomato paste and stock or water and season with salt and pepper. Reduce the heat to low and simmer, covered, for 1 hour until reduced and thickened, stirring occasionally. If the sauce is too thin, remove the lid and simmer until reduced and thickened. Cool slightly. Cook the spinach with just the water clinging to the leaves in a covered saucepan for 1 minute, or until wilted.

Meanwhile, to make the white sauce, put the starch in a saucepan, add a little of the milk and mix to a smooth paste. Add the remaining milk, onion slice and nutmeg. Stir constantly over medium heat until the sauce boils and thickens. Reduce the heat and simmer for 1 minute. Remove the onion. Stir in the cheeses, then mix until smooth.

Preheat the oven to 350°F. Arrange one-third of the lasagna sheets over the base of a 16-cup rectangular ovenproof dish. Spoon over half the beef, then cover with half the spinach. Cover with another layer of pasta and spoon over the remaining beef. Cover with the remaining spinach, then the remaining pasta. Spread over the white sauce. Bake for 30 minutes, or until golden. Rest for 5 minutes before slicing.

nutrition per serving (8): Energy 426 Cal; Fat 14.3 g; Saturated fat 6.6 g; Protein 26 g; Carbohydrate 49 g; Fiber 4.2 g; Cholesterol 57 mg

THREE BEAN CHILI WITH RICE

2 tsp canola or olive oil
1 large onion, finely chopped
3 garlic cloves, crushed
2 tbsp ground cumin
1 tbsp ground cilantro
1 tsp ground cinnamon
1 tsp chili powder
15 oz canned diced tomatoes
1⅔ cups vegetable stock GF (Basics)
15 oz tin chickpeas GF, drained and rinsed
15 oz canned red kidney beans GF, drained and rinsed

15 oz canned cannellini (white) beans GF, drained and rinsed
2 tbsp tomato paste GF
2 tsp sugar
2 cups basmati rice, rinsed and drained

PREP TIME: 20 MINUTES
COOKING TIME: 35 MINUTES
SERVINGS 4

Heat the oil in a large frying pan and cook the onion over medium–low heat for 5 minutes, or until golden, stirring frequently. Reduce the heat, add the garlic, cumin, cilantro, cinnamon and chili powder, then stir for 1 minute.

Add the tomatoes, stock, chickpeas, kidney beans and cannellini beans and combine with the onion mixture. Bring to a boil, then simmer for 20 minutes, stirring occasionally. Add the tomato paste and sugar and season to taste with salt and freshly ground black pepper. Simmer for a further 5 minutes.

Meanwhile, put the rice and 4 cups water in a saucepan and bring to a boil over medium heat. Reduce the heat to low, cover with a lid and cook for 20 minutes, or until the rice is tender. Remove from the heat and leave to stand, covered, for 5 minutes. Serve with the bean chili.

HINTS:
- It's a good idea to check the label of canned beans to ensure the manufacturer has not used additives or preservatives that contain gluten.
- Top the dish with a little yogurt or grated cheddar cheese, if you like; if you use pre-grated cheddar cheese, check the packet to make sure it doesn't contain gluten.

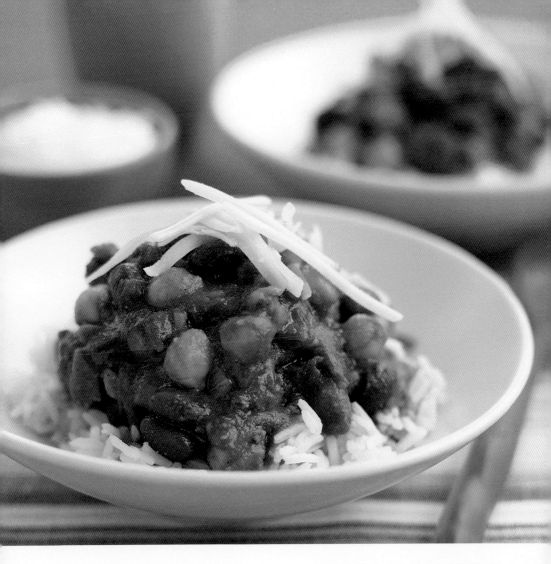

THIS VEGETARIAN MEAL IS A GREAT CHOICE FOR PEOPLE WITH DIABETES OR A HIGH BLOOD CHOLESTEROL LEVEL—IT'S LOW GI, LOW IN FAT AND HIGH IN SOLUBLE FIBER.

nutrition per serving: Energy 697 Cal
Fat 7.4 g
Saturated fat 0.9 g
Protein 30.4 g
Carbohydrate 129.4 g
Fiber 21.9 g
Cholesterol 0 mg

TUNA KEBABS WITH CHICKPEA TOMATO SALSA

THIS IS A FILLING, LOW-GI MEAL THAT PROVIDES SOME HEALTHY OMEGA-3 FAT (GOOD FOR THE HEART, BRAIN AND EYES, AND FOR REDUCING INFLAMMATION).

SALSA

2 tsp olive oil

2–3 small red chilies, seeded and finely chopped

3–4 garlic cloves, crushed

1 red onion, finely chopped

3 tomatoes, seeded and chopped

3 tbsp dry white wine or water

26 oz chickpeas GF, drained and rinsed

3 tbsp chopped oregano

4 tbsp chopped parsley

about 2 lbs tuna fillet

canola or olive oil spray

lemon wedges, to serve

PREP TIME: 20 MINUTES

COOKING TIME: 20 MINUTES

SERVINGS 4

To make the salsa, heat the oil in a large saucepan, add the chili, garlic and onion and stir for 5 minutes, or until softened. Add the tomato and wine or water. Cook over low heat for 10 minutes, or until the mixture is soft, pulpy and the liquid has evaporated. Stir in the chickpeas, oregano and parsley. Season with salt and freshly ground black pepper.

Meanwhile, trim the tuna and cut into 1½ in cubes. Heat a cast-iron grill. Thread the tuna onto eight metal skewers, lightly spray with the oil, then cook, turning, for 3 minutes. Do not overcook or the tuna will fall apart. Serve with the salsa and lemon wedges.

HINTS:
- If you are using wooden skewers, soak them in water for 30 minutes before use.
- Check the can of chickpeas to ensure no gluten-containing ingredients have been added.

nutrition per serving: Energy 534 Cal; Fat 20 g; Saturated fat 6.6 g; Protein 70.6 g; Carbohydrate 17 g; Fiber 7.7 g; Cholesterol 90 mg

CHILI CON POLLO

THIS EASY RECIPE IS THE CHICKEN LOVER'S VERSION OF CHILI CON CARNE.
IF YOU PREFER, YOU CAN MAKE THE MEATIER VERSION BY REPLACING THE
CHICKEN WITH AN EQUAL WEIGHT OF GROUND LEAN BEEF.

2 tsp olive oil

1 onion, finely chopped

about 1 lb lean ground chicken

1–2 tsp mild chili powder

15 oz canned diced tomatoes

2 tbsp tomato paste (concentrated
    purée) GF

15 oz canned red kidney beans GF, drained
    and rinsed

2 cups basmati rice, drained and rinsed

4 tbsp chopped parsley

1 cup low-fat plain yogurt

PREP TIME: 10 MINUTES
COOKING TIME: 1 HOUR
SERVINGS 4

Heat the oil in a large saucepan. Add the onion and cook over medium heat for 3 minutes, or until soft. Increase the heat and add the chicken. Cook until browned, breaking up any lumps with a wooden spoon.

Add the chili powder and cook for 1 minute. Add the tomato, tomato paste and ½ cup water and stir well. Bring to a boil, then reduce the heat and simmer for 30 minutes. Stir in the kidney beans and heat through. Season to taste with salt and freshly ground black pepper.

Meanwhile, put the rice and 4 cups water in a saucepan and bring to a boil over medium heat. Reduce the heat to low, cover with a lid and cook for 20 minutes, or until the rice is tender. Remove from the heat and leave to stand, covered, for 5 minutes.

Sprinkle the chili con pollo with the parsley and serve with the yogurt and rice.

HINTS:
- Many people with long-standing untreated celiac disease become iron deficient. If this applies to you, make the recipe with beef mince to increase your iron stores.
- When using canned beans always check the ingredient list to ensure no additives or preservatives that contain gluten have been added.

nutrition per serving: 683 Cal; Fat 13.8 g; Saturated fat 3.6 g; Protein 40.3 g; Carbohydrate 98 g; Fiber 7.5 g; Cholesterol 116 mg

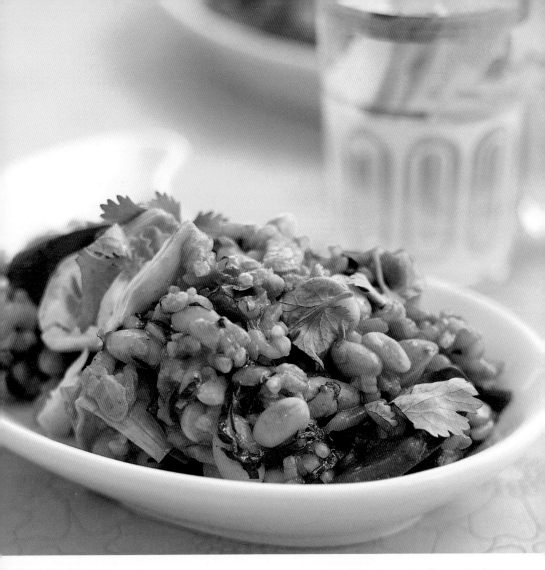

IT'S WORTH THE EFFORT IT TAKES TO COOK THIS HEARTY DISH BECAUSE THE RESULT IS SO DELICIOUS. THE VARIETY OF FOODS IN THIS MEAL MAKES IT HIGHLY NUTRITIOUS—IT'S A GREAT SOURCE OF FOLATE, FIBER AND VARIOUS ANTIOXIDANTS.

nutrition per serving: Energy 366 Cal

Fat 5.2 g

Saturated fat 0.9 g

Protein 17.6 g

Carbohydrate 57.1 g

Fiber 11.6 g

Cholesterol 0 mg

VEGETARIAN PAELLA

1 cup dried haricot beans
¼ tsp saffron threads
2 tsp olive oil
1 onion, diced
1 red pepper, cut into thin strips
5 garlic cloves, crushed
1¼ cups paella or arborio rice
1 tbsp sweet paprika
½ tsp mixed spice
3 cups vegetable stock GF (Basics)
15 oz canned diced tomatoes

1½ tbsp tomato paste GF
2⅓ cups fresh or frozen soybeans
3½ oz Swiss chard, shredded
15 oz canned artichoke hearts in brine, drained and rinsed
4 tbsp chopped cilantro leaves

PREP TIME: 20 MINUTES +
  OVERNIGHT SOAKING
COOKING TIME: 40 MINUTES
SERVINGS 6

Put the haricot beans in a large bowl, cover with cold water and leave to soak overnight. Drain and rinse well.

Place the saffron threads in a small frying pan over medium–low heat. Dry-fry, shaking for 1 minute, or until darkened. Remove from the heat and, when cool, crumble into a small bowl. Pour in ½ cup warm water and allow to steep.

Heat the oil in a large paella pan or frying pan. Add the onion and pepper and cook over medium–high heat for 5 minutes, or until the onion softens. Stir in the garlic and cook for 1 minute. Reduce the heat and add the drained beans, rice, paprika, mixed spice and season with salt. Stir to coat. Add the saffron water, stock, tomatoes and tomato paste and bring to a boil. Cover, reduce the heat and simmer for 20 minutes.

Stir in the soybeans, Swiss chard and artichoke hearts and cook, covered, for 8 minutes, or until all the liquid is absorbed and the rice and beans are tender. Turn off the heat and leave for 5 minutes. Stir in the cilantro just before serving.

HINTS:
- Always check the label of commercial stocks to ensure there are no ingredients that contain gluten. Better yet, make your own.
- Top with some grated cheese or plain yogurt for extra calcium—if you're using pre-grated cheese, make sure no flour has been added by the manufacturer.

HUNGARIAN-STYLE PORK AND LENTIL STEW

THIS MEAL IS LOW IN FAT, LOW GI, AND A GOOD SOURCE OF IRON, ZINC AND B-GROUP VITAMINS, INCLUDING VITAMIN B12.

2 tsp olive oil

2 onions, chopped

about 1 lb lean diced pork

2 tsp sweet paprika

1 tsp hot paprika

½ tsp dried thyme

2 tbsp tomato paste GF

1 tsp brown sugar

3 tbsp red lentils

1½ cups beef stock GF (Basics)

1 tomato

2 cups basmati rice, rinsed and drained

2 tbsp low-fat plain yogurt

PREP TIME: 20 MINUTES

COOKING TIME: 1 HOUR 5 MINUTES

SERVINGS 4

Heat the olive oil in a large, deep saucepan over high heat. Add the onion, pork and paprika and stir for 3–4 minutes, or until browned.

Add the thyme, tomato paste, sugar, lentils and stock and season with salt and freshly ground black pepper. Bring to a boil, reduce the heat to very low and cook, covered, for 20 minutes, stirring occasionally to prevent sticking. Uncover and cook for 15–20 minutes, or until thickened.

Remove from the heat and set aside for 10 minutes. To prepare the tomato, cut it in half and scoop out the seeds. Slice the flesh into thin strips.

Meanwhile, put the rice and 4 cups water in a saucepan and bring to a boil over medium heat. Reduce the heat to low, cover with a lid and cook for 20 minutes, or until the rice is tender. Remove from the heat and leave to stand, covered, for 5 minutes. Just before serving, stir the yogurt into the stew. Scatter with tomato. Serve with the rice and a salad.

HINT:
• If you have diabetes and you want to serve this stew with gluten-free pasta or noodles instead of basmati rice, choose a gluten-free pasta with a lower GI, such as a soy-based pasta, or serve with fresh rice noodles.

nutrition per serving: Energy 592 Cal; Fat 6.5 g; Saturated fat 1.6 g; Protein 41.1 g; Carbohydrate 91.8 g; Fiber 5.1 g; Cholesterol 119 mg

LAMB CASSEROLE WITH BEANS

THIS CASSEROLE MAKES A GREAT MEAL ON A COLD WINTER'S NIGHT—IT'S WARM AND NOURISHING. COOK DOUBLE PORTIONS SO YOU CAN FREEZE THE LEFTOVERS TO USE AS QUICK WEEKDAY MEALS.

1½ cups dried borlotti or red kidney beans

about 2 lb lean boned leg of lamb

2 tsp olive oil

1¾ oz low-fat bacon slices ^{GF}, chopped

1 large onion, chopped

2 garlic cloves, crushed

1 large carrot, peeled and chopped

2 cups red wine

1 tbsp tomato paste ^{GF}

1½ cups beef stock ^{GF} (Basics)

2 large sprigs of rosemary

2 sprigs of thyme

PREP TIME: 25 MINUTES +
    OVERNIGHT SOAKING

COOKING TIME: 2¼ HOURS

SERVINGS 6

Put the beans in a large bowl, cover with water and leave to soak overnight. Drain well.

Preheat the oven to 315°F. Trim any fat from the lamb and cut into bite-sized cubes.

Heat the oil in a large flameproof casserole dish over high heat and brown the lamb in two batches for 2 minutes. Remove all the lamb from the dish and set aside. Add the bacon and onion to the casserole dish. Cook over medium heat for 3 minutes, or until the onion is soft. Add the garlic and carrot and cook for 1 minute, or until fragrant.

Return the lamb and any juices to the pan, increase the heat to high and add the wine. Bring to a boil and cook for 2 minutes. Add the beans, tomato paste, stock, rosemary and thyme, bring to a boil, then cover and cook in the oven for 2 hours, or until the meat is tender. Stir occasionally during cooking and skim off any fat from the surface. Season with salt and freshly ground black pepper and remove the herb sprigs before serving.

HINTS:
- Serve with some gluten-free pasta or bread.
- Gluten can be a hidden additive in many foods, such as bacon, tomato paste and stock. Always check the labels carefully.

nutrition per serving: Energy 460 Cal; Fat 13.1 g; Saturated fat 5.3 g; Protein 51 g; Carbohydrate 23 g; Fiber 10.7 g; Cholesterol 113 mg

HERB-CRUSTED LAMB ROAST WITH VEGETABLES

6 large carrots, peeled and cut into ¾
    in pieces on the diagonal
canola or olive oil spray
2 tbsp Dijon mustard GF
2 tbsp finely chopped flat-leaf (Italian)
    parsley
1 tsp finely chopped thyme
1 tsp finely chopped sage
3 garlic cloves, crushed
10½ oz pieces lamb rump or mini lamb
    roasts, trimmed

8–10 small new potatoes
1 cup vegetable stock GF (Basics)
4 cups frozen peas, thawed
2 tbsp mint

PREP TIME: 20 MINUTES
COOKING TIME: 1 HOUR
SERVINGS 4

Preheat the oven to 400°F. Spray the carrots with the oil, season well and place into a large roasting pan (you will be adding the lamb pieces halfway through cooking). Cook in the oven for 1 hour, or until golden and soft.

Place the mustard, parsley, thyme, sage and two of the crushed garlic cloves in a bowl. Mix well to combine and add the lamb pieces. Thoroughly coat with the mixture and add to the carrots in the roasting pan 30 minutes before it is due to be ready.

Meanwhile, cook the new potatoes in a large saucepan of boiling water for 12 minutes, or until tender. Drain.

In a small saucepan over high heat, bring the vegetable stock to the boil with the remaining crushed garlic clove. Add the peas and cook for 3 minutes. Remove from the heat and strain, reserving the stock. Put the peas, mint and reserved stock in a food processor. Blend until smooth, then season to taste.

Remove the lamb from the oven and allow to rest, covered, on a board for 5 minutes before slicing across the grain. Divide among four plates and serve with the boiled potatoes, pea and mint purée and roasted carrots.

HINT:
• You should be able to find a gluten-free mustard in the supermarket—just check the label.

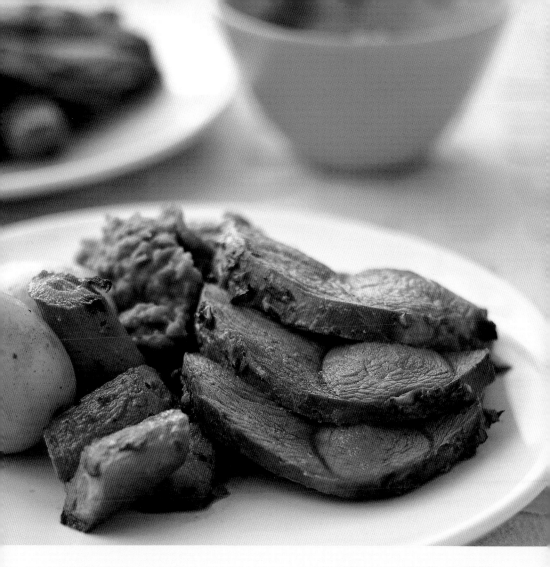

CANCEL YOUR DINNER
RESERVATIONS—YOU CAN
ENJOY THIS RESTAURANT-STYLE
FOOD AT HOME WITHOUT
HAVING TO CHECK IF IT'S FREE
OF GLUTEN. SERVE IT TO
FAMILY AND FRIENDS.

nutrition per serving: Energy 479 Cal

Fat 8.4 g

Saturated fat 2.7 g

Protein 45.5 g

Carbohydrate 46.7 g

Fiber 16.5 g

Cholesterol 102 g

95

CHICKEN WITH SNOW PEAS, SPROUTS AND NOODLES

THIS QUICK GLUTEN-FREE MEAL IS A GREAT RECIPE TO ADD TO YOUR COLLECTION OF FAVOURITE WEEKDAY RECIPES. IT TAKES LITTLE TIME TO PREPARE AND COOK AND GIVES YOU A NUTRITIOUS, FILLING MEAL.

10½ oz dried mung bean vermicelli
about 1 lb boneless, skinless chicken breast
2 tsp canola or olive oil
1 onion, thinly sliced
3 kaffir lime leaves, shredded
1 red pepper, sliced
½ cup snow peas, trimmed
3 tbsp lime juice
½ cup tamari GF

3 tbsp snow pea (mangetout) sprouts, trimmed
2 tbsp chopped cilantro leaves

PREP TIME: 15 MINUTES +
  10 MINUTES SOAKING
COOKING TIME: 30 MINUTES
SERVINGS 4

Put the noodles in a large bowl and cover with warm water. Soak for 10 minutes, or until they are translucent. Drain. Transfer to a saucepan of boiling water and cook for 10 minutes, or until tender. Rinse under cold water and drain.

Meanwhile, trim the chicken and cut into thin slices. Heat a wok over medium heat, add the oil and swirl to coat. Add the onion and kaffir lime leaves and stir-fry for 3–5 minutes, or until the onion begins to soften. Remove from the wok. Add the chicken in batches and cook for a further 4 minutes, or until lightly browned. Remove from the wok and set aside. Reheat the wok between batches.

Return the onion mixture and all the chicken to the wok, add the pepper and snow peas and continue to cook for 2–3 minutes. Stir in the lime juice, tamari and 2 tablespoons water and cook for 1–2 minutes, or until the sauce reduces slightly. Add the noodles and toss through the mixture to warm through. Add the sprouts and cilantro and cook until the sprouts have wilted slightly.

HINT:
• Use the chicken, tamari and lime juice as a base, then add vegetables and herbs to taste. For example, use asparagus instead of snow peas, or mint instead of cilantro.

nutrition per serving: Energy 505 Cal; Fat 9.3 g; Saturated fat 2.3 g; Protein 30.9 g; Carbohydrate 71.3 g; Fiber 2.1 g; Cholesterol 82 mg

MIXED BEANS AND PEPPER STIR-FRY

THIS DISH TAKES LESS THAN 30 MINUTES TO MAKE AND CAN BE SERVED AS A SIDE DISH OR AS A VEGETARIAN MAIN MEAL. IT'S LOW GI AND RICH IN FIBER, ANTIOXIDANTS AND FOLATE.

2 tsp canola or olive oil
2 garlic cloves, crushed
1 red onion, cut into thin wedges
1 red pepper, cut into short, thin strips
1 yellow pepper, cut into short, thin strips
15 oz canned chickpeas GF, drained and rinsed
15 oz canned red kidney beans GF, drained and rinsed
1 tsp brown sugar
2 tbsp balsamic vinegar

3 tbsp lime juice
9 oz cherry tomatoes, halved
1 cucumber, chopped
3 tbsp chopped cilantro leaves
butter lettuce leaves, to serve

PREP TIME: 15 MINUTES
COOKING TIME: 10 MINUTES
SERVINGS 6

Heat a wok until very hot, add the oil and swirl to coat. Add the garlic, onion and red and yellow pepper strips and stir-fry over medium heat for 2–3 minutes. Remove from the wok and set aside.

Add the chickpeas and kidney beans to the wok, stir in the brown sugar and balsamic vinegar and toss for 2–3 minutes, or until the liquid has reduced by half. Add the lime juice and toss until well combined.

Using two wooden spoons, stir in the cherry tomatoes, cucumber, cilantro and the onion and capsicum mixture. Stir-fry briefly until heated through and thoroughly mixed. Put a couple of lettuce leaves on each plate and spoon the stir-fry onto the leaves to serve.

HINTS:
- Even though most canned legumes don't contain gluten it's a good idea to check the ingredient list to ensure the manufacturer has not added any gluten-containing additives or preservatives.
- Serve the stir-fry with basmati rice or quinoa instead of lettuce leaves for a more balanced low-GI vegetarian meal.

nutrition per serving: Energy 114 Cal; Fat 2.8 g; Saturated fat 0.3 g; Protein 6.4 g; Carbohydrate 15.3 g; Fiber 6.1 g; Cholesterol 0 mg

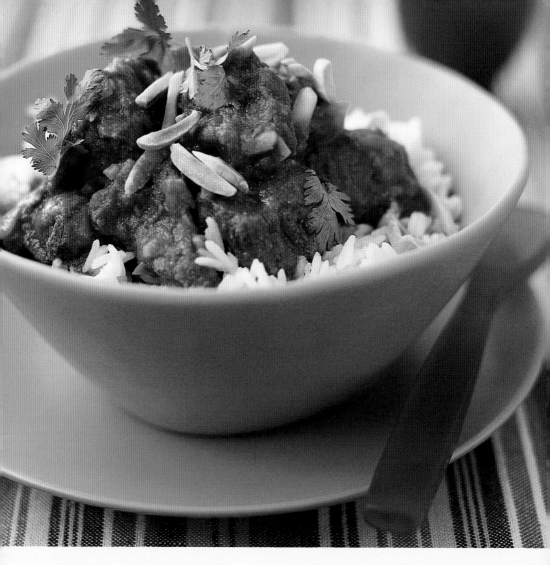

IF YOU CAN'T BE SURE THAT YOUR
LOCAL INDIAN RESTAURANT HAS
GLUTEN-FREE DISHES AVAILABLE,
THEN A HOME-MADE CURRY IS THE
SAFEST OPTION. THIS LAMB CURRY
IS A GOOD SOURCE OF IRON, ZINC
AND B-GROUP VITAMINS.

nutrition per serving: Energy 555 Cal
Fat 15.2 g
Saturated fat 5.3 g
Protein 44.6 g
Carbohydrate 59.5 g
Fiber 3.4 g
Cholesterol 114 mg

ROGAN JOSH

about 2 lbs lean boned leg of lamb

2 tsp canola or olive oil

2 onions, chopped

½ cup low-fat plain yogurt

1 tsp chili powder

1 tbsp ground cilantro

2 tsp ground cumin

1 tsp ground cardamom

1 tsp ground turmeric

½ tsp ground cloves

3 garlic cloves, crushed

1 tbsp grated fresh ginger

15 oz canned diced tomatoes

1 tsp salt

3 tbsp slivered almonds

2 cups basmati rice, rinsed and drained

1 tsp garam masala

chopped cilantro leaves, to serve

PREP TIME: 25MINUTES

COOKING TIME: 2 HOURS

SERVINGS 6

Trim the lamb of any fat or sinew and cut into small cubes. Heat the oil in a large heavybased saucepan, add the onion and cook, stirring, for 5 minutes, or until soft. Stir in the yogurt, chili powder, cilantro, cumin, cardamom, turmeric, cloves, garlic and ginger. Add the tomato and salt and simmer for 5 minutes.

Add the lamb and stir until coated. Cover and cook over low heat, stirring occasionally, for 1–1½ hours, or until the lamb is tender. Uncover and simmer until the liquid thickens.

Meanwhile, toast the almonds in a dry frying pan over medium heat for 3–4 minutes, shaking the pan gently, until the nuts are golden brown. Remove from the pan at once to prevent them burning. Put the rice and 4 cups water in a saucepan and bring to a boil over medium heat. Reduce the heat to low, cover with a lid and cook for 20 minutes, or until the rice is tender. Remove from the heat and leave to stand, covered, for 5 minutes.

Add the garam masala to the curry and mix through well. Sprinkle the slivered almonds and cilantro leaves over the top and serve with the rice.

HINTS:
- This curry is delicious served the next day, after the flavors have had time to develop more fully.
- Serve with plain gluten-free poppadoms—cook them in a microwave, so they contain less fat and are ready in a flash. Other traditional Indian side dishes also make refreshing accompaniments to this meal (such as cucumber raita, tomato and onions, and bananas in lemon juice and grated coconut).

TANDOORI FISH CUTLETS

THE SPICES ADD COLOR, FLAVOR AND VALUABLE MINERALS TO THIS LOW-GI DISH. MARINATING THE FISH OVERNIGHT SAVES PREPARATION TIME THE NEXT DAY.

4 firm white fish cutlets
3 tbsp lemon juice
1 onion, finely chopped
2 garlic cloves, crushed
1 tbsp grated fresh ginger
1 red chili
1 tbsp garam masala
1 tsp paprika
¼ tsp salt

2 cups low-fat plain yogurt
2 cups basmati rice, rinsed and drained

PREP TIME: 20 MINUTES +
  OVERNIGHT MARINATING
COOKING TIME: 30 MINUTES
SERVINGS 4

Pat the fish cutlets dry with paper towels and arrange in a shallow non-metallic dish. Drizzle the lemon juice over the fish and turn to coat the cutlets with the juice.

To make the marinade, blend the onion, garlic, ginger, chili, garam masala, paprika and salt in a blender until smooth. Transfer to a bowl and stir in the yogurt. Spoon the marinade over the fish and turn the fish to coat thoroughly. Cover and refrigerate overnight.

Put the rice and 4 cups water in a saucepan and bring to a boil over medium heat. Reduce the heat to low, cover with a lid and cook for 20 minutes, or until the rice is tender. Remove from the heat and leave to stand, covered, for 5 minutes.

Meanwhile, heat a broiler or barbecue . Remove the cutlets from the marinade and allow any excess to drip off. Cook the cutlets under the grill or on the barbecue for 3–4 minutes on each side, or until the fish flakes easily when tested with a fork. Serve with the rice.

HINTS:
- Try blue eye, snapper or warehou.
- This is delicious served with extra yogurt and baby spinach leaves or a cooling cucumber raita.

nutrition per serving: Energy 653 Cal; Fat 8.2 g; Saturated fat 4.1 g; Protein 53.9 g; Carbohydrate 89 g; Fiber 2.7 g; Cholesterol 142 mg

CILANTRO BEEF WITH NOODLES

THIS IS THE PERFECT RECIPE FOR A QUICK WEEKDAY MEAL. MARINATE THE MEAT OVERNIGHT, SO ALL YOU HAVE TO DO THE NEXT DAY IS QUICKLY PREPARE THE REST OF THE INGREDIENTS, THEN STIR-FRY.

4 garlic cloves, finely chopped
1 tbsp finely chopped fresh ginger
1 large handful cilantro, stems and leaves, chopped
3 tsp canola or olive oil
about 1 lb lean beef rump steak
14 oz fresh rice noodles
1 red onion, thinly sliced
½ red pepper, thinly sliced
½ green pepper, thinly sliced

2 tbsp lime juice
2 tbsp tamari GF
1 large handful cilantro leaves, extra

PREP TIME: 20 MINUTES +
  2 HOURS MARINATING
COOKING TIME: 20 MINUTES
SERVINGS 4

To make the marinade, combine the garlic, ginger, cilantro and 2 teaspoons of the oil in a large non-metallic bowl. Trim the beef, then cut into thin strips across the grain. Add to the marinade and toss to coat. Cover with plastic wrap and refrigerate for 2 hours or overnight.

Put the rice noodles in a large heatproof bowl, cover with boiling water and soak for 8 minutes, or until softened. Separate gently and drain.

Heat a wok until very hot and spray with canola or olive oil. Add the meat in three batches and stir-fry for 2–3 minutes, or until the meat is just cooked. Remove all the meat from the wok and keep it warm. Reheat and respray the wok between batches.

Heat the remaining 1 teaspoon oil in the wok, add the onion and cook over medium heat for 3–4 minutes, or until slightly softened. Add the pepper slices and cook, tossing constantly, for a further 3–4 minutes, or until slightly softened.

Return all the meat to the wok along with the lime juice, tamari, 2 tablespoons water and extra cilantro. Add the noodles. Toss well, then remove from the heat and season well with salt and freshly ground black pepper.

HINT:
• Tamari is usually wheat free but check the label to ensure it is gluten free.

nutrition per serving: Energy 406 Cal; Fat 10 g; Saturated fat 2.8 g; Protein 32.6 g; Carbohydrate 44.3 g; Fiber 2.2 g; Cholesterol 80 mg

GREEK-STYLE CALAMARI

STUFFING

2 tsp olive oil

2 spring onions (scallions), sliced

1½ cups cold, cooked basmati rice

4 tbsp pine nuts

4 tbsp finely chopped dried apricots

2 tbsp chopped parsley

2 tsp finely grated lemon zest

1 egg, lightly beaten

about 1 lb cleaned squid tubes

SAUCE

4 large ripe tomatoes

2 tsp olive oil

1 onion, finely chopped

1 garlic clove, crushed

3 tbsp good-quality red wine

1 tbsp chopped oregano

PREP TIME: 30 MINUTES

COOKING TIME: 35 MINUTES

SERVINGS: 4–6

Preheat the oven to 315°F. To make the stuffing, mix together the oil, spring onion, rice, pine nuts, apricots, parsley and lemon zest in a bowl. Add enough egg to moisten all the ingredients.

Wash the squid tubes and pat dry inside and out with paper towels. Three-quarters fill each squid tube with the stuffing. Secure the ends with toothpicks or skewers. Place in a single layer in a casserole dish.

To make the sauce, begin by peeling the tomatoes. Score a cross in the base of each one. Cover with boiling water for 30 seconds, then plunge into cold water. Drain and peel away the tomato skin from the cross. Chop the flesh. Heat the oil in a frying pan. Add the onion and garlic and cook over low heat for 2 minutes, or until the onion is soft. Add the tomato, wine and oregano and bring to a boil. Reduce the heat, cover with a lid and cook over low heat for 10 minutes.

Pour the hot sauce over the squid, cover and bake for 20 minutes, or until the squid is tender. Remove the toothpicks before cutting into thick slices for serving. Spoon the sauce over just before serving.

HINT:
• You will need to cook ½ cup raw basmati rice for this recipe.

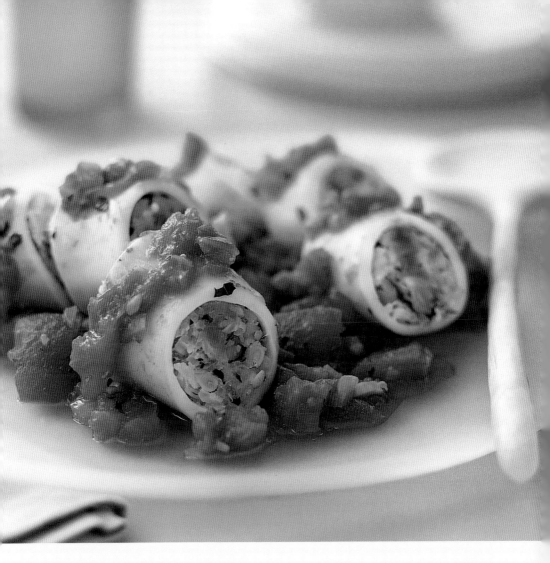

TAKE A TRIP TO THE COAST OF
THE MEDITERRANEAN WITH THIS
TASTY DISH. IT'S MUCH MORE
NUTRITIOUS THAN DEEP-FRIED
COMMERCIAL CALAMARI—IT'S LOW
GI AND PROVIDES GOOD AMOUNTS
OF THE MINERALS IRON, ZINC,
IODINE AND SELENIUM.

nutrition per serving (6): Energy 346 Cal
Fat 13.2 g
Saturated fat 1.8 g
Protein 33.4 g
Carbohydrate 21.7 g
Fiber 3.9 g
Cholesterol 363 mg

SPRING VEGETABLE RISOTTO

WELCOME THE RETURN OF SPRING WITH THIS DELICIOUS RISOTTO. YOU CAN STIR IN SOME FRESHLY COOKED CHICKEN PIECES BEFORE SERVING FOR A MORE SUBSTANTIAL MEAL WITH MORE PROTEIN, IRON AND ZINC.

9 oz cherry tomatoes

3 unpeeled garlic cloves

3 sprigs of thyme

canola or olive oil spray

7 cups chicken or vegetable stock GF
   (Basics)

2 tsp olive oil

1 onion, finely chopped

2 cups arborio rice

6 oz asparagus, trimmed and cut into
   ¾ in pieces

6 oz baby carrots, halved on the diagonal

¾ cup frozen peas, thawed

2 tbsp chopped mint

2 tbsp chopped basil

2 tbsp chopped flat-leaf (Italian) parsley

4 tbsp freshly grated parmesan cheese

PREP TIME: 20 MINUTES

COOKING TIME: 30 MINUTES

SERVINGS: 4

Preheat the oven to 350°F. Toss the tomatoes in a glass or ceramic ovenproof dish with the unpeeled garlic cloves and thyme. Spray with the oil. Season with salt and freshly ground black pepper, then bake, uncovered, for 30 minutes, or until the tomatoes are soft but still whole.

Meanwhile, pour the stock into a saucepan and bring to a boil. Reduce the heat and keep the stock at a gentle simmer. Heat the oil in a heavy-based saucepan over medium heat, add the onion and cook, stirring, for 6–7 minutes, or until the onion has softened. Add the rice and stir through for 1 minute, or until well coated.

Add ½ cup of the hot stock. Cook over medium heat, stirring constantly, until most of the stock has been absorbed. Continue adding the stock, ½ cup at a time, stirring constantly. After 15 minutes, add the asparagus and carrot, then continue adding the remaining stock until it has all been absorbed and the rice is creamy and tender. Stir through the peas, herbs and parmesan. Season to taste.

Serve the risotto in individual serving bowls topped with the roasted cherry tomatoes and drizzled with any juices from the cooked tomatoes.

nutrition per serving: Energy 553 Cal; Fat 6.8 g; Saturated fat 2.3 g; Protein 17.7 g; Carbohydrate 100.8 g; Fiber 7.9 g; Cholesterol 26 mg

CRUNCHY COATED CHICKEN

IF YOU MISS REGULAR BATTERED OR CRUMBED FRIED CHICKEN, THEN THIS RECIPE IS FOR YOU: IT'S A LOWER FAT, GLUTEN-FREE VERSION. IT CAN BE SERVED WARM OR COLD AND MAKES A GOOD ADDITION TO A PICNIC HAMPER.

½ **cup gluten-free plain**
  (all-purpose) flour
2 eggs
1 cup rice bran
2–3 tbsp poppy seeds
4–5 chicken pieces,
  skin removed
canola or olive oil spray

CHIVE YOGURT
½ **cup low-fat plain yogurt** GF
2 tbsp snipped chives

PREP TIME: 20 MINUTES +
  30 MINUTES REFRIGERATION
COOKING TIME: 30 MINUTES
SERVINGS: 4

Preheat the oven to 400°F. Lightly grease a baking tray.

Put the flour in a shallow bowl. Mix the eggs with 2 tablespoons water in a separate bowl and mix the bran, poppy seeds and a little salt in a third bowl. Dust the chicken pieces lightly with the flour. Dip them in the combined egg and water, then roll in the bran mixture, pressing the mixture on firmly. Put the chicken pieces on the prepared tray and refrigerate for 30 minutes to firm the coating.

Spray the chicken all over with oil spray. Bake for about 30 minutes, or until golden brown and cooked through when tested.

Meanwhile, to make the chive yogurt, combine the yogurt and chives in a small bowl, then season to taste with salt.

Serve the chicken hot or cold with the chive yogurt.

HINT:
• Serve with a salad and potato wedges.

nutrition per serving: Energy 642 Cal; Fat 27.1 g; Saturated fat 6.5 g; Protein 66.9 g; Carbohydrate 27.9 g; Fiber 8.1 g; Cholesterol 313 mg

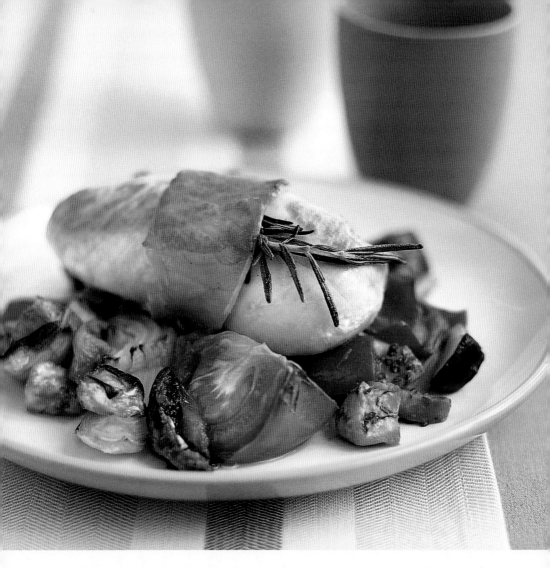

THIS COLORFUL MEAL IS FULL OF THE FLAVORS OF THE MEDITERRANEAN. IT PROVIDES GOOD AMOUNTS OF PROTEIN, IRON, ZINC AND ANTIOXIDANTS. SERVE WITH RICE, QUINOA, GLUTEN-FREE PASTA OR BREAD.

nutrition per serving: Energy 359 Cal
Fat 12.7 g
Saturated fat 3.5 g
Protein 50.6 g
Carbohydrate 8.6 g
Fiber 5.4 g
Cholesterol 132 mg

CHICKEN WITH BAKED EGGPLANT AND TOMATO

1 red pepper
1 eggplant
3 tomatoes
7 oz large button mushrooms
1 onion
canola or olive oil spray
1½ tbsp tomato paste GF
½ cup chicken stock GF (Basics)
3 tbsp dry white wine
2 low-fat bacon slices GF

4 boneless, skinless chicken breasts
4 small sprigs of rosemary

PREP TIME: 30 MINUTES
COOKING TIME: 1½ HOURS
SERVINGS: 4

Preheat the oven to 400°F. Cut the pepper and eggplant into bite-sized pieces. Cut the tomatoes into quarters, the mushrooms in half and the onion into thin wedges. Mix the vegetables together in a roasting tin. Spray with the oil and bake for 1 hour, or until starting to brown and soften, stirring once.

Mix together the tomato paste, stock and wine, then pour into the roasting tin and roast the vegetables for a further 10 minutes, or until the sauce has thickened.

Meanwhile, cut the bacon in half lengthways. Wrap a strip around each chicken breast and secure it underneath with a toothpick. Poke a sprig of fresh rosemary underneath the bacon. Heat a non-stick frying pan over medium heat. Spray with the oil. Cook the chicken for 2–3 minutes on each side, or until golden on both sides. Cover and cook for 10–15 minutes, or until the chicken is cooked through. Remove the toothpicks. Serve the chicken on a bed of the vegetables.

HINTS:
- Always check the ingredient list of commercial stocks because they often contain gluten.
- Gluten can be added in the preserving process of meats such as bacon, so check the ingredient list before you buy.

SEAFOOD PASTA

THIS PASTA DISH IS A GREAT CHOICE FOR ACTIVE PEOPLE—A SINGLE SERVING PROVIDES PLENTY OF CARBOHYDRATE FOR ENERGY AND GOOD AMOUNTS OF MANY VITAMINS AND MINERALS.

1 tbsp olive oil

1 large onion, cut into thin wedges

2 garlic cloves, crushed

2¾ oz button mushrooms, thinly sliced

3 ripe tomatoes, roughly chopped

28 oz canned diced tomatoes

1 tbsp tomato paste GF

1 tsp sugar

1 tsp freshly ground black pepper

3 tbsp capers, rinsed, drained and chopped

8 medium raw shrimp, peeled and deveined

8 scallops, trimmed

2 small cleaned squid tubes, cut into rings

1 large handful flat-leaf (Italian) parsley, finely chopped

1 handful basil, shredded

about 1 lb gluten-free fettuccine or other pasta

freshly grated parmesan cheese, to serve (optional)

PREP TIME: 15 MINUTES
COOKING TIME: 30 MINUTES
SERVINGS: 4–6

Heat the olive oil in a large, deep, heavy-based saucepan. Add the onion and garlic and cook for 2 minutes, or until softened. Add the mushrooms, tomatoes, tomato paste, sugar, pepper, capers and 1 cup water. Bring to a boil, then reduce the heat and simmer for 20 minutes. Stir in the shrimps, scallops and squid, then cook for a further 2–3 minutes until the seafood is just cooked. Just before serving, stir in the parsley and basil.

Meanwhile, cook the pasta in a large saucepan of boiling salted water for 10 minutes, or according to the instructions, until just tender. Drain well and return to the saucepan. Toss through the sauce. Divide into bowls and serve with the grated parmesan cheese, if you like.

nutrition per serving (6): Energy 446 Cal; Fat 5.1 g; Saturated fat 0.9 g; Protein 20.6 g; Carbohydrate 75.8 g; Fiber 6.2 g; Cholesterol 110 mg

GINGER CHILI FISH CUTLETS WITH CILANTRO RICE

THIS ASIAN-STYLE MEAL IS A GREAT CHOICE FOR PEOPLE WHO ARE WATCHING THEIR WEIGHT.

2 cups basmati rice, rinsed and drained
4 firm white fish cutlets
2 in piece of fresh ginger, shredded
2 garlic cloves, chopped
2 tsp chopped red chili
2 tbsp chopped cilantro stems and leaves
3 spring onions (scallions), thinly sliced
cilantro leaves, chopped, extra
3 tbsp lime juice

1 tbsp fish sauce GF
2 tsp honey

PREP TIME: 20 MINUTES
COOKING TIME: 30 MINUTES
SERVINGS: 4

Put the rice and 4 cups water in a saucepan and bring to a boil over medium heat. Reduce the heat to low, cover with a lid and cook for 20 minutes, or until the rice is tender. Remove from the heat and leave to stand, covered, for 5 minutes.

Meanwhile, cook the fish. Line a large bamboo steamer basket with baking paper or banana leaves. Arrange the fish in the basket and top with the ginger, garlic, chili and cilantro stems and leaves. Cover with a lid and steam over a wok or large saucepan of boiling water for 8–10 minutes, without letting the basket touch the water. Sprinkle the spring onion over the fish. Cover and steam for a further 30 seconds, or until the fish flakes easily with a fork.

Stir the extra cilantro leaves into the rice. Divide the rice onto serving plates. Top with the fish and pour over the combined lime juice, fish sauce and honey.

HINTS:
- Try snapper, sea bass or blue eye.
- There are many brands of gluten-free fish sauce available.

nutrition per serving: Energy 534 Cal; Fat 3.2 g; Saturated fat 1.1 g; Protein 39.7 g; Carbohydrate 84.1 g; Fiber 1.6 g; Cholesterol 96 mg

RICE-CRUMBED FISH WITH WEDGES

2 eggs
2 tbsp milk
4 tbsp gluten-free all-purpose flour
1 cup rice crumbs
4 boneless white fish fillets
canola or olive oil spray
lettuce or salad leaves, to serve
chutney GF (Basics), to serve

WEDGES
3–4 large all-purpose potatoes, peeled and
cut into wedges
canola or olive oil spray

PREP TIME: 20 MINUTES
COOKING TIME: 50 MINUTES
SERVINGS: 4

Preheat the oven to 425°F. Line two large baking trays with sheets of baking paper.

Combine the eggs and milk in a shallow bowl. Put the flour in a shallow dish and season with salt and pepper. Put the rice crumbs in a separate shallow dish. Dip the fish in the flour, followed by the egg mixture and, lastly, the rice crumbs. Lay the crumbed fish in a single layer on one of the lined trays. Refrigerate until required.

Put the potato wedges in a large bowl and sprinkle with salt. Spray the wedges with oil, then toss to coat. Spread over the second lined tray.

Bake the potato wedges for 30 minutes, turning once. Put the wedges on the lower shelf of the oven. Remove the fish from the fridge, then spray both sides of the fish lightly with oil. Add the fish to the top shelf and cook for 20 minutes, or until the fish is cooked and the wedges are crispy. Serve the fish with the wedges, lettuce and chutney.

HINT:
- It can be hard to find gluten-free versions of commercially available chutneys, relishes and sauces, so why not make your own instead?

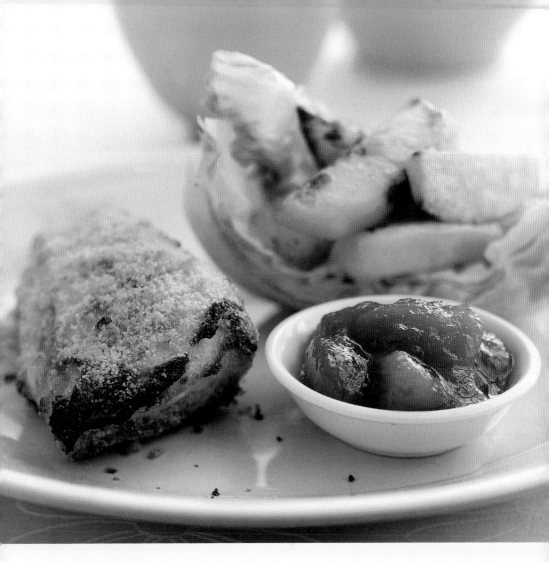

YOU DON'T NEED TO AVOID FISH AND CHIPS WHEN YOU'RE ON A GLUTENFREE DIET—JUST MAKE YOUR OWN GLUTEN-FREE VERSION. OVEN-BAKING THE FISH AND CHIPS MAKES THIS VERSION MUCH LOWER IN FAT THAN THE DEEP-FRIED VARIETY.

nutrition per serving: Energy 492 Cal
Fat 9.1 g
Saturated fat 2.4 g
Protein 42.7 g
Carbohydrate 56.1 g
Fiber 4 g
Cholesterol 188 mg

SIRLOIN STEAKS WITH ROASTED PEPPERS AND GREEN OLIVE SALAD

IF YOU HAVE AN IRON DEFICIENCY, TRY THIS MEAL. IT'S A GREAT SOURCE OF WELL-ABSORBED IRON AND CAN BE ENJOYED BY THE WHOLE FAMILY.

8–10 small new potatoes
1 red pepper, seeded and quartered
½ green beans, trimmed and halved
about 1 lb lean sirloin steak, cut into 4
fillets or 4 x 4 oz fillet steaks
1 cup red wine
2 tbsp balsamic vinegar
1 tbsp brown sugar
10 small thyme leaves
4 handfuls mixed salad leaves

½ cup green olives in brine, pitted and lightly squashed
1 tbsp baby capers, rinsed and drained (optional)

PREP TIME: 20 MINUTES
COOKING TIME: 25 MINUTES
SERVINGS: 4

Put the potatoes in a saucepan of boiling water. Cook for 12 minutes, or until tender, then drain, refresh and cut in half. Set aside.

Meanwhile, preheat a grill or broiler to medium. Roast the pepper until the skin blackens and blisters. Set aside in a plastic bag for 5 minutes, then peel away the skin and slice the flesh into thin strips. Blanch the beans for 2 minutes in a saucepan of boiling water. Drain and refresh.

Pat the meat dry with paper towels. Lightly brush a non-stick frying pan with oil and heat to very hot. Add the meat and cook for 2–3 minutes on each side, or until cooked to your liking. Remove from the pan, cover with foil and set aside while preparing the sauce.

Add the wine, vinegar, sugar and half of the thyme leaves to the frying pan. Bring to a boil, stirring continuously. Boil until reduced by about one-third. Set aside until just warm.

Toss together the salad leaves, pepper and beans in a large bowl. Divide the salad leaves equally onto four large plates. Scatter over the potatoes, olives and capers, if using. Cut the fillets into ½ in thick slices and arrange on top of the salad. Drizzle over the dressing and garnish with the remaining thyme leaves.

nutrition per serving: Energy 407 Cal; Fat 9.5 g; Saturated fat 3.6 g; Protein 31.8 g; Carbohydrate 34.3 g; Fiber 5.8 g; Cholesterol 72 mg

SPAGHETTI BOLOGNESE

THIS GLUTEN-FREE VERSION OF THE TRADITIONAL RECIPE IS A REAL CROWD PLEASER AND IS A GREAT CHOICE FOR A HEALTHY WEEKDAY MEAL. IT IS ALSO DELICIOUS SERVED AS LEFTOVERS THE NEXT DAY.

1 tbsp canola or olive oil

1 onion, chopped

2 large garlic cloves, crushed

1 celery stalk, diced

1 carrot, peeled and diced

3¼ oz button mushrooms, finely chopped

about 1 lb lean ground beef

1 tsp dried oregano

1 cup red wine

1 cup beef stock GF (Basics)

28 oz canned diced tomatoes

2 tbsp tomato paste GF

16 oz gluten-free spaghetti

freshly grated parmesan cheese, to serve

2 tbsp chopped basil

PREP TIME: 20 MINUTES

COOKING TIME: 1 ½ HOURS

SERVINGS: 4

Heat the oil in a large, non-stick saucepan. Add the onion and cook, stirring occasionally, for 3 minutes. Add the garlic, celery, carrot and mushroom and cook for a further 2 minutes. Add the minced beef and cook over high heat for 5 minutes, or until cooked, breaking up any lumps with the back of a spoon. Add the oregano and wine and cook for 3–4 minutes, or until most of the liquid has evaporated.

Add the stock, tomatoes and tomato paste and season with salt and pepper. Reduce the heat to low and simmer, covered, for 1 hour, stirring occasionally to prevent it from catching on the bottom. If the sauce is too thin, remove the lid and simmer until reduced and thickened. Cool slightly.

Meanwhile, cook the spaghetti in a large saucepan of boiling, salted water for 10 minutes, or according to the packet instructions, until tender. Drain well. Toss the spaghetti with the sauce and serve with the parmesan and basil.

HINTS:
- You can serve regular or gluten-free spaghetti with this bolognese sauce, if you need to cater to different family members. Just make sure that you cook the two types of pasta in separate saucepans and drain in separate colanders.
- Serve with a mixed leaf salad dressed with balsamic vinegar.

nutrition per serving: Energy 653 Cal; Fat 14.7 g; Saturated fat 4.2 g; Protein 35.4 g; Carbohydrate 78.6 g; Fiber 6.5 g; Cholesterol 64 mg

113

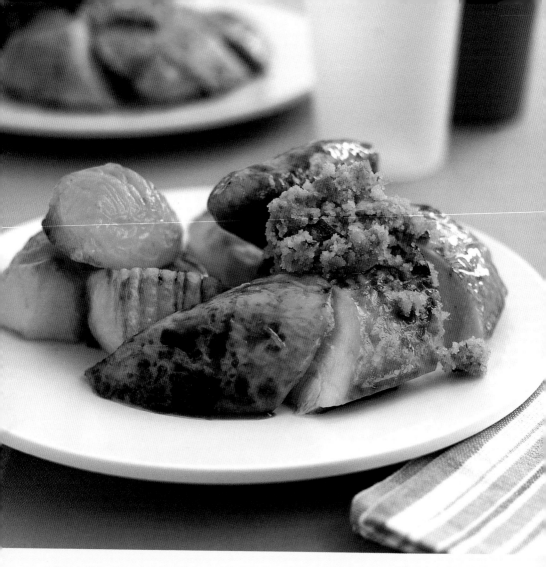

BORED WITH REGULAR ROAST CHICKEN? TRY THIS VERSION FOR A CHANGE. SERVE WITH A VARIETY OF STEAMED VEGETABLES FOR A SATISFYING MEAL. REMEMBER TO TAKE THE SKIN OFF THE CHICKEN BEFORE YOU EAT IT, IF YOU'RE WATCHING YOUR WEIGHT.

nutrition per serving: Energy 603 Cal
Fat 38.6 g
Saturated fat 12.6 g
Protein 45.7 g
Carbohydrate 19 g
Fiber 0.5 g
Cholesterol 245 mg

ROAST CHICKEN WITH STUFFING

about 3½ lbs whole chicken
2 tsp canola or olive oil
1 tbsp golden syrup or honey

PUMPKIN AND BREADCRUMB STUFFING
1 tsp butter
2 spring onions (scallions), thinly sliced
1 garlic clove, crushed

1 cup fresh gluten-free breadcrumbs
½ cup finely grated butternut squash

PREP TIME: 30 MINUTES
COOKING TIME: 1½ HOURS
SERVINGS: 4

Preheat the oven to 350°F. Lightly oil a roasting pan. To prepare the chicken, remove the neck, rinse out the cavity with cold water and pat dry with paper towels.

To make the stuffing, melt the butter in a small frying pan over medium heat, add the spring onions and garlic and cook, stirring, until softened. Combine the breadcrumbs and pumpkin in a bowl. Add the spring onion mixture and season with salt and pepper. Spoon the stuffing into the chicken cavity. Close the cavity using poultry pins or by tying the legs together with string. Tuck the neck flap underneath.

Combine the oil and golden syrup or honey in a small saucepan and heat until warm, then brush all over the chicken. Sprinkle lightly with salt and pepper.

Put the chicken in the roasting pan and roast for 1¼–1½ hours, basting every 15 minutes with the pan juices. Cover with oiled foil if the chicken starts to over-brown. It is cooked when the juices run clear when a skewer is inserted into the thickest part of the thigh. Rest for 10 minutes before carving.

HINTS:
- Make your own gluten-free breadcrumbs by placing gluten-free bread slices in a food processor and blend until crumbs form—you'll need about 3 average slices of gluten-free bread without crusts.
- You can experiment with the stuffing. For example, you can replace the breadcrumbs with some cooked quinoa or buckwheat.
- Serve the chicken with roast potatoes and a variety of steamed vegetables.

FRESH TOMATO AND OLIVE PASTA

THIS PASTA SAUCE GOES EQUALLY WELL WITH GLUTEN-FREE OR REGULAR PASTA SO IT'S EASY TO PREPARE SEPARATE MEALS FOR THE GLUTEN-TOLERANT MEMBERS OF YOUR FAMILY. JUST REMEMBER TO USE A SEPARATE POT.

3–4 vine-ripened tomatoes, finely chopped
1 small red onion, finely chopped
2 garlic cloves, finely chopped
½ cup chopped pitted green olives in brine
3 tbsp capers, rinsed, drained and chopped
1 tsp dried oregano
3 tbsp olive oil
1 tbsp white wine vinegar
16 oz gluten-free rigatoni

14 oz canned fava or lima beans GF, drained and rinsed
1 handful oregano

PREP TIME: 15 MINUTES +
  1 HOUR STANDING
COOKING TIME: 10 MINUTES
SERVINGS: 4

Combine the tomatoes, onion, garlic, olives, capers and dried oregano in a bowl. Whisk together the oil and vinegar in a small bowl, then toss through the tomato mixture. Season with salt and pepper. Cover and set aside for at least 1 hour to allow the flavors to develop.

Meanwhile, cook the pasta in a large saucepan of boiling salted water for 10 minutes, or according to the packet instructions, until just tender. Drain and return to the saucepan. Toss the tomato mixture and butter beans through the hot pasta. Divide among four bowls, then garnish with the oregano leaves.

HINTS:
- You can use any type of gluten-free pasta shapes.
- If you prefer, omit the beans or replace them with soybeans, chickpeas or lentils, but remember to check the label for any gluten-containing additives.

nutrition per serving: Energy 641 Cal; Fat 15.7 g; Saturated fat 2.4 g; Protein 10.7 g; Carbohydrate 110.4 g; Fiber 7.9 g; Cholesterol 0 mg

HAMBURGERS

YOU DON'T NEED TO GIVE UP FUN FOODS LIKE HAMBURGERS JUST BECAUSE YOU'RE ON A GLUTEN-FREE DIET. IN FACT, THE MEAT IN HAMBURGERS IS AN EXCELLENT SOURCE OF IRON, ZINC AND VITAMIN B12.

about 1 lb lean ground beef
4 spring onions (scallions), thinly sliced
3 tbsp snipped chives
1 garlic clove, crushed
1 egg
1¼ cups gluten-free puffed rice, finely crushed
canola or olive oil, for frying
12 slices of gluten-free bread

2 tbsp butter
½ head lettuce, shredded
chutney GF or tomato sauce GF (Basics)

PREP TIME: 30 MINUTES
COOKING TIME: 20 MINUTES
MAKES 6

Combine the beef, spring onions, chives, garlic, egg, puffed rice and 3 tablespoons water in a large bowl. Season with salt and pepper. Using your hands, knead the mixture until well combined. Divide the mixture into six portions. Roll into balls, then flatten into patties. Heat the oil in a large frying pan over medium heat, add the patties and cook for about 4–6 minutes on each side, or until cooked through and lightly browned.

Use a large cookie cutter to cut the bread into rounds. Otherwise, leave the slices square. Spread one side of each bread slice with butter and broil, butter side up, for 1–2 minutes, or until crisp and golden brown.

Place a patty and lettuce between two slices of toasted bread. Serve topped with a dollop of chutney or tomato sauce.

HINTS:
- Use a gluten-free bread that toasts well and won't go soggy when you add the hamburger. If you try different brands of gluten-free bread on a regular basis, you can work out which ones toast better than others. Some will have a lighter texture than others. A stronger bread works best with a hamburger.
- These burgers are great for kids because they are fairly plain, perfect for fussy eaters. You can make them more interesting by adding other ingredients. For instance, hide a little grated carrot and zucchini in the beef patties to secretly get children to eat some more vegetables—add a little beaten egg to help bind the mixture. A slice of low-fat cheddar cheese in the burger is another good addition as it will provide extra calcium.

nutrition per serving: Energy 413 Cal; Fat 13.3 g; Saturated fat 6.5 g; Protein 24.2 g; Carbohydrate 48.4 g; Fiber 1.5 g; Cholesterol 96 mg

GREEK-STYLE LAMB

about 1 lb lean lamb fillets

1 tsp olive oil

1 large red onion, sliced

3 zucchini, thinly sliced

7 oz cherry tomatoes, halved

3 garlic cloves, crushed

½ cup pitted black olives in brine, drained
   and halved

2 tbsp lemon juice

2 tbsp oregano

⅔ cup crumbled low-fat feta cheese

4 tbsp pine nuts, lightly toasted

PREP TIME: 20 MINUTES
COOKING TIME: 10 MINUTES
SERVINGS: 4

Trim the lamb, then cut across the grain into thin strips. Heat a large frying pan until hot and lightly brush with oil. Add the lamb in small batches and cook each batch over high heat for 1–2 minutes, or until browned. Remove all the lamb from the pan.

Heat the oil in the pan, then add the onion and zucchini. Cook, stirring, over high heat for 2 minutes, or until just tender. Add the cherry tomatoes and garlic. Cook for 1–2 minutes, or until the tomatoes have just softened. Return the meat to the pan and stir over high heat until heated through.

Remove the pan from the heat. Add the olives, lemon juice and oregano and toss until well combined. Sprinkle with crumbled feta cheese and pine nuts before serving.

HINT:
• Serve with gluten-free bread rolls or corn tortillas and a mixed green salad.

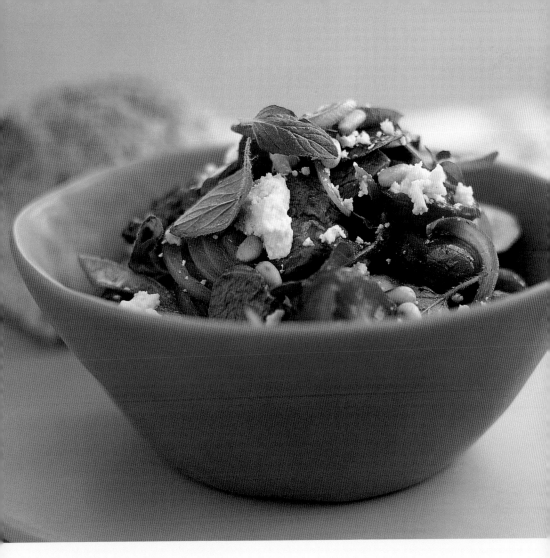

THIS DISH IS SURE TO IMPRESS YOUR FRIENDS AND FAMILY, BUT YOU DON'T NEED TO SAVE IT FOR SPECIAL OCCASIONS—IT MAKES A GOOD WEEKDAY MEAL. YOU CAN ALSO SERVE THIS DISH WITH RICE INSTEAD OF GLUTEN-FREE BREAD, IF YOU PREFER.

nutrition per serving: Energy 451 Cal

Fat 20 g

Saturated fat 5.5 g

Protein 34.6 g

Carbohydrate 31.1 g

Fiber 7.2 g

Cholesterol 78 mg

119

PORK AND CABBAGE NOODLE STIR-FRY

STIR-FRIES ARE A GREAT WAY TO MAKE HEALTHY MEALS WHEN YOU'RE SHORT OF TIME—JUST HAVE ALL THE INGREDIENTS READY BEFORE YOU BEGIN.

SAUCE
1½ tbsp fish sauce GF
4 tbsp tamari GF
1½ tbsp brown sugar

14 oz thin rice stick noodles
2 tsp canola or olive oil
1 onion, finely chopped
2 garlic cloves, finely chopped
1–2 long red chilies, seeded and finely chopped

about 1 lb lean ground pork
1 large carrot, peeled and grated
1 zucchini, grated
3 cups thinly shredded cabbage
1 large handful cilantro leaves

PREP TIME: 15 MINUTES
COOKING TIME: 10 MINUTES
SERVINGS: 4

Combine the sauce ingredients in a small bowl, stirring to dissolve the sugar. Place the noodles in a large bowl and cover with boiling water. Set aside for 4 minutes, or until softened. Drain well. Use scissors to cut the noodles into shorter lengths.

Heat the oil in a wok. Add the onion, garlic, chili and pork and stir-fry for 4 minutes, or until browned and cooked. Break up any lumps as you cook.

Stir in the carrot, zucchini and cabbage and continue to stir-fry for a further 2–3 minutes, or until the vegetables are just cooked. Stir through the noodles, then the sauce ingredients and cilantro leaves.

HINTS:
- Always check the ingredient list on bottles of tamari and fish sauce as they can be hidden sources of gluten.
- If you prefer spicy food, leave the seeds in the chili.

nutrition per serving: Energy 552 Cal; Fat 12.5 g; Saturated fat 3.5 g; Protein 35.3 g; Carbohydrate 71.7 g; Fiber 5.9 g; Cholesterol 75 mg

FISH STEAKS WITH MUSHROOMS

THIS ASIAN-STYLE RECIPE WILL APPEAL TO FISH LOVERS AS IT CAN BE USED
TO PREPARE SEVERAL DIFFERENT TYPES OF FISH (SNAPPER, SWORDFISH,
COD, SALMON AND HALIBUT, TO NAME A FEW).

2 tbsp tamari GF
1 tbsp canola or olive oil
grated zest and juice of 1 lemon
2 tbsp Chinese rice wine or dry sherry
4 x 7 oz snapper steaks
1 tsp sesame oil
5½ oz fresh shiitake mushrooms, sliced
2 spring onions (scallions), sliced

PREP TIME: 15 MINUTES +
   4 HOURS MARINATING
COOKING TIME: 35 MINUTES
SERVINGS: 4

Mix the tamari, oil, lemon zest and juice and rice wine or sherry together in a bowl. Put the fish steaks in a shallow, glass or ceramic ovenproof dish in which they fit snugly in a single layer. Pour the marinade over the fish and turn them once so both sides are coated. Cover and refrigerate for at least 4 hours, or overnight, turning the fish over in the marinade a couple of times.

Remove the fish from the fridge and let it return to room temperature. Preheat the oven to 350°F.

Heat the sesame oil in a frying pan over medium heat and, when hot, add the mushrooms. Cook and stir for 3–4 minutes, or until starting to soften. Add the spring onions, then stir and remove the pan from the heat.

Sprinkle the mushroom and onion mixture over the fish and bake, covered with a lid or foil, for 25–30 minutes, or until the fish is opaque and firm to the touch.

HINTS:
• Although tamari is usually wheat free, it is not always gluten free.
• Chinese rice wine (sometimes labelled Shaoxing) is available at Asian food stores. If you can't find it, use dry sherry instead.
• Serve with rice or gluten-free noodles and steamed green vegetables or salad.

nutrition per serving: Energy 279 Cal; Fat 8.1 g; Saturated fat 1.8 g; Protein 42.2 g; Carbohydrate 6 g; Fiber 1.1 g; Cholesterol 122 mg

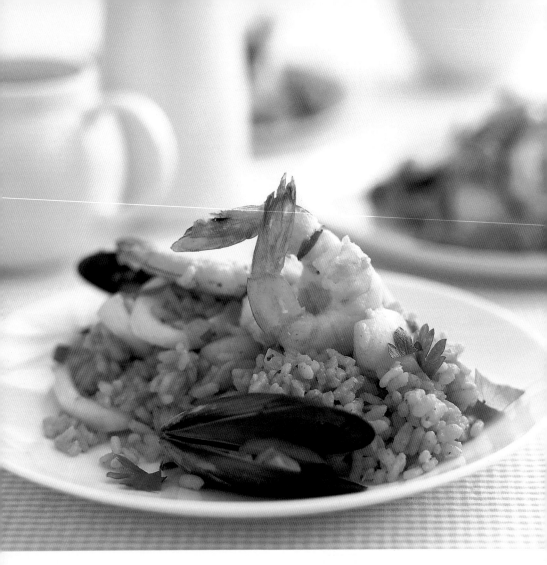

A SEAFOOD BUFFET IN ONE MEAL—
THIS DISH COMBINES A DELICIOUS
MIX OF SEAFOOD WITH A HERBED
RISOTTO FOR A FILLING, NUTRITIOUS
MEAL. IT'S A GOOD SOURCE OF
PROTEIN AND MINERALS INCLUDING
IRON, ZINC, IODINE AND SELENIUM.

nutrition per serving: Energy 616 Cal
Fat 5.8 g
Saturated fat 1.4 g
Protein 40.6 g
Carbohydrate 92.6 g
Fiber 1.3 g
Cholesterol 233 mg

SEAFOOD RISOTTO

12 black mussels

½ cup dry white wine

6 cups fish or chicken stock (Basics)

1 small pinch of saffron threads

2 tsp olive oil

8 raw shrimp, peeled and deveined, tails
    intact

8 scallops, trimmed with coral intact

3 small squid tubes, cleaned and cut
    into rings

1 onion, finely chopped

2 garlic cloves, crushed

2 cups arborio rice

2 tbsp chopped flat-leaf (Italian) parsley

PREP TIME: 25 MINUTES

COOKING TIME: 45 MINUTES

SERVINGS: 4

Scrub the mussels with a stiff brush and remove the beards. Discard any broken mussels or any that don't close when tapped. Place the mussels in a heavy-based saucepan with the wine and cook, covered, over high heat, for 3–4 minutes, or until the mussels have just opened. Remove any that have not opened and discard. Strain and reserve the liquid and set the mussels aside.

Combine the mussel liquid, stock and saffron in a saucepan, then cover and keep at a low simmer. Heat 1 teaspoon of the oil in a non-stick frying pan over medium–high heat. Add the shrimps and cook until they just turn pink. Remove to a plate, then cook the scallops and squid in batches for 1–2 minutes, or until lightly golden. Remove and set aside with the mussels and shrimps.

Heat the remaining teaspoon of oil in a heavy-based saucepan, then add the onion and garlic. Reduce the heat to low and cook for 5–6 minutes, or until soft and translucent. Add the rice and stir until coated. Add ½ cup of the hot stock, stirring constantly with a wooden spoon until absorbed. Continue adding ½ cup of liquid at a time, stirring constantly, until all the liquid is absorbed. This should take about 25 minutes. Stir through the seafood and parsley. Season to taste and serve immediately.

HINTS:
- If you're using a commercial stock, make sure it doesn't contain gluten.
- Serve with a mixed leaf salad dressed with balsamic vinegar.

123

THAI CHICKEN SALAD

ENJOY THIS DELICIOUS, FRAGRANT SALAD WHEN THE WEATHER IS WARM. IT'S LIGHT AND REFRESHING SO IS THE PERFECT CHOICE. YOU CAN SPICE IT UP WITH RED CHILI, IF YOU LIKE.

3½ oz dried rice vermicelli
about ½ lb ground chicken
7 oz canned water chestnuts, drained and
  chopped
2 tbsp fish sauce GF
2 tbsp lime juice
1 lemon grass stem, white part only,
finely chopped

3 spring onions (scallions), thinly sliced
3 tbsp chopped Thai basil
3 tbsp chopped mint

PREP TIME: 15 MINUTES +
  10 MINUTES SOAKING
COOKING TIME: 5 MINUTES
SERVINGS: 4

Put the dried rice vermicelli in a large bowl. Pour over enough boiling water to cover and soak for 10 minutes, or until tender. Drain and pat dry.

Put the chicken, water chestnuts, fish sauce, lime juice, lemon grass and 3 tablespoons water in a frying pan and stir over medium heat for 5 minutes, or until the chicken is cooked. Set aside to cool. Transfer to a bowl and add the spring onions, basil, mint and vermicelli. Toss well to combine. Serve immediately.

HINTS:
- Fish sauce can be a hidden source of gluten in Asian food so always check the label.
- Thai basil is distinguishable by its purple stems and flowers. If you can't find it, use normal basil instead.

nutrition per serving: Energy 191 Cal; Fat 5.2 g; Saturated fat 1.4 g; Protein 13.7 g; Carbohydrate 21 g; Fiber 1.8 g; Cholesterol 55 mg

SPICED LAMB WITH DAL AND YOGURT

THIS DISH IS A REAL PLEASURE TO MAKE—THE SPICES WILL FILL YOUR KITCHEN WITH DELICIOUS AROMAS THAT WILL STIMULATE YOUR APPETITE.

3 tsp cumin seeds

1 tbsp cilantro seeds

1 tsp garam masala

2 x 9 oz lean lamb loin fillets

2 cups long-grain white rice

low-fat plain yogurt GF**, to serve**

DAL

¾ heaping cup red lentils

¼ tsp ground turmeric

3 cups chicken stock GF **(Basics)**

2 tsp brown mustard seeds

2 tsp ground cumin

1 onion, finely chopped

3 garlic cloves, crushed

½ tsp chili flakes

3 tbsp chopped cilantro leaves

PREP TIME: 20 MINUTES + 2 HOURS MARINATING

COOKING TIME: 1 HOUR

SERVINGS: 4

Put the cumin and cilantro seeds and garam masala in a small, dry frying pan and toast for 1 minute, or until fragrant. Put in a spice grinder, or use a mortar and pestle, and grind until coarse. Season, then rub onto the lamb. Cover and refrigerate for 2 hours.

Bring 4 cups water to a boil in a large saucepan. Stir in the rice. Cover the pan, reduce the heat and simmer for 20 minutes. Uncover, stir and stand for 5 minutes.

To make the dal, put the lentils and turmeric in a saucepan, cover with the stock and bring to a boil over high heat. Reduce the heat to low and simmer for 20 minutes, stirring occasionally, or until the lentils are tender.

Spray a non-stick saucepan with canola or olive oil, then heat over high heat. Add the mustard seeds and cumin and cook for 1 minute, or until the mustard seeds begin to pop. Add the onion and cook for 2–3 minutes, or until softened. Add the garlic and chili and cook for 30 seconds. Add the lentil mixture and cilantro, reduce the heat to low and cook for 5 minutes, stirring, or until reduced and thickened. Keep warm.

Lightly spray a cast-iron grill with oil and heat over high heat. Add the lamb and cook for 4–5 minutes on each side. Cover and stand for 5 minutes. Cut into ½ in slices on the diagonal. Divide the rice and dal onto four plates and top with the lamb. Serve with yogurt.

nutrition per serving: Energy 724 Cal; Fat 10.9 g; Saturated fat 2.8 g; Protein 48.8 g; Carbohydrate 103.7 g; Fiber 9.8 g; Cholesterol 85 mg

125

CHICKEN AND LEEK PIE

about ¾ lb boneless, skinless chicken
breast
2 tbsp butter
1 leek, washed and thinly sliced
1 celery stalk, thinly sliced
4 slices of low-fat bacon ^{GF}, thinly sliced
2 tsp pure maize cornstarch ^{GF}
¾ cup low-fat milk
1 egg yolk
1 small handful parsley, chopped

1 cup firmly packed grated low-fat cheddar
cheese ^{GF}
1 quantity gluten-free shortcrust pastry
(Basics)

PREP TIME: 30 MINUTES +
20 MINUTES STANDING
COOKING TIME: 55 MINUTES
SERVINGS: 4

To make the filling, put the chicken in a saucepan and cover with cold water. Slowly bring to a boil, then simmer for 2 minutes. Turn off the heat, cover and set aside 20 minutes.

Heat the butter in a medium frying pan. Add the leek, celery and bacon. Cook, stirring occasionally for 5 minutes over low heat until the leek is soft. In a small bowl combine the cornstarch with a little of the milk. Mix until smooth. Add the remaining milk and egg yolk. Pour over the leek mixture. Stir over a low heat for 2–3 minutes until thickened. Season with salt and pepper.

Shred the chicken with a fork, then stir it into the leek mixture. Transfer to a plate to cool completely, then stir in the parsley. Preheat the oven to 400°F.

Lightly grease a 9 in fluted tart pan, then line it with the prepared pastry. Trim to fit the tin. The pastry is soft and malleable so just fill any tears and cracks if necessary. Reserve the leftover dough.

Place the tin on a baking tray. Cover the pastry with a sheet of baking paper and half fill with baking beads or rice. Bake for 10 minutes. Remove the beads and paper and bake for a further 10–15 minutes, or until lightly browned. Fill any cracks with small amounts of reserved pastry. Bake for a further 2 minutes to set. Remove from the oven and cool completely. Reduce the oven temperature to 350°F.

Fill the cooled pastry with the cooled filling. Scatter the cheese over the top. Bake for 20 minutes until cooked and the pastry is golden brown.

HINT:
• Serve with a mixed salad or steamed vegetables.

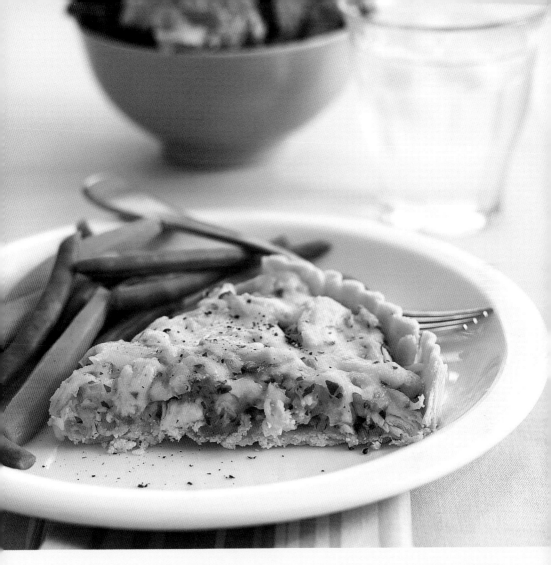

PIES ARE A GREAT COMFORT
FOOD, PARTICULARLY IN WINTER.
THIS RECIPE WILL HELP
CONVINCE NEWLY DIAGNOSED
CELIACS THAT A GLUTEN-FREE
DIET DOESN'T HAVE TO BE A
BLAND, BORING AFFAIR.

nutrition per serving: Energy 649 Cal

Fat 31.8 g

Saturated fat 19.2 g

Protein 42.2 g

Carbohydrate 48.4 g

Fiber 1.8 g

Cholesterol 249 mg

BEEF AND NOODLE SALAD

SPICE UP YOUR WEEKLY MENU WITH THIS ASIAN-STYLE SALAD, WHICH IS QUICK AND EASY TO MAKE. THE MIXTURE OF HERBS ADDS LOTS OF FLAVOR AND AROMA AS WELL AS FOLATE AND ANTIOXIDANTS.

DRESSING
2 tbsp finely chopped lemon grass, white
    part only
1 small red chili
3 tbsp tamari GF
3 tbsp lime juice
1 tbsp fish sauce GF
1 tbsp brown sugar
1 tsp grated fresh ginger

about 1 lb lean sirloin steak
7 oz cellophane (bean thread) noodles
1 cucumber
1 small red onion

4 ripe Roma (plum) tomatoes
1 tbsp thinly shredded fresh ginger
1 cup bean sprouts, trimmed
1 handful mint, torn
1 handful basil, torn
1 handful cilantro leaves

PREP TIME: 15 MINUTES +
   15 MINUTES MARINATING
COOKING TIME: 10 MINUTES
SERVINGS: 4

Bruise the lemon grass using a mortar and pestle or a heavy object such as a rolling pin. Seed and finely chop the chili. Combine the dressing ingredients using a mortar and pestle or in a bowl and stir to dissolve the sugar. Put 1 tablespoon of the dressing in a shallow non-metallic dish with the meat. Coat the meat with the dressing and marinate for at least 15 minutes. Set aside the remaining dressing.

Spray a non-stick frying pan or cast-iron pan with oil. Heat the oil until very hot. Add the steak and cook for 2–3 minutes on each side, or until cooked as desired. Remove and set aside for 5 minutes, then slice thinly.

Place the noodles in a large bowl and cover with boiling water. Set aside for 4 minutes, drain well and refresh under cold water. Use scissors to cut into short lengths.

Cut the cucumber in half lengthways, then thinly slice on the diagonal. Cut the onion into thin wedges. Cut the tomatoes into quarters. Put into a large bowl with the rest of the ingredients. Toss together gently with the remaining dressing so everything is covered. Serve immediately.

nutrition per serving: Energy 415 Cal; Fat 8.9 g; Saturated fat 3.5 g; Protein 29.7 g; Carbohydrate 51.7 g; Fiber 3 g; Cholesterol 72 mg

WARM SHRIMP AND SCALLOP STIR-FRY

THIS DISH IS QUITE SIMPLE TO MAKE—JUST HAVE ALL OF THE INGREDIENTS MEASURED AND READY TO GO BEFORE YOU FIRE THE WOK UP.

2 cups basmati rice, rinsed and drained

2 tsp five-spice

1–2 small red chilies, seeded and finely chopped

2–3 garlic cloves, crushed

2 tsp sesame oil

about 1 lb raw shrimps, peeled and deveined, tails intact

10½ oz scallops, trimmed, with coral intact

7 oz asparagus, trimmed and cut into short lengths

5½ oz snow peas, trimmed

2¾ cups arugula

2 tbsp tamari GF

2 tbsp lemon juice

1 tbsp mirin

2 tsp honey

6 spring onions (scallions), sliced

1 tbsp chopped cilantro leaves

1 tbsp sesame seeds, toasted

PREP TIME: 30 MINUTES +
 10 MINUTES MARINATING
COOKING TIME: 35 MINUTES
SERVINGS: 4

Put the rice and 4 cups water in a saucepan and bring to a boil over medium heat. Reduce the heat to low, cover with a lid and cook for 20 minutes, or until the rice is tender. Remove from the heat and leave to stand, covered, for 5 minutes.

Meanwhile, combine the five-spice, chili, garlic and sesame oil in a large non-metallic bowl. Add the shrimps and scallops and toss to coat. Cover with plastic wrap and refrigerate for at least 10 minutes.

Blanch the asparagus and snow peas. Drain and plunge into a bowl of iced water, then drain again. Arrange on four plates with the arugula. Combine the tamari, lemon juice, mirin and honey in a small bowl.

Heat a wok over high heat, add the seafood and spring onions in batches and cook for 3–4 minutes, or until cooked through, reheating the wok between batches. Remove from the wok and set aside. Add the tamari–lemon sauce and cilantro to the wok, then bring to a boil. Cook over high heat for 1–2 minutes. Return the seafood to the wok and toss well. Divide among the plates and sprinkle with the sesame seeds. Serve with the rice.

nutrition per serving: Energy 545 Cal; Fat 5.8 g; Saturated fat 0.8 g; Protein 33.2 g; Carbohydrate 88.7 g; Fiber 4.7 g; Cholesterol 118 mg

DESSERTS

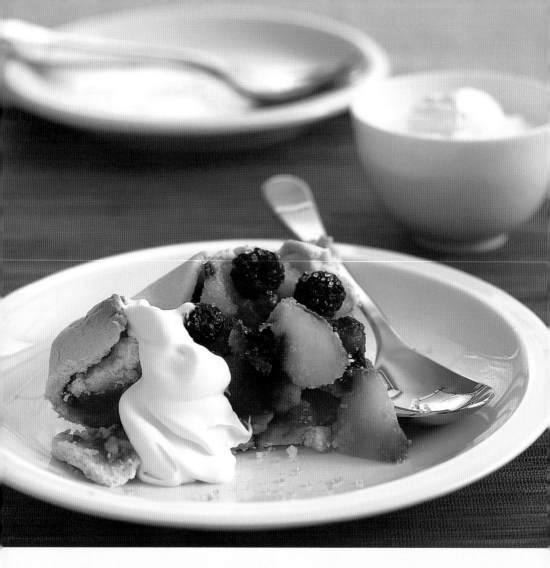

FOR A COMFORTING WINTER
DESSERT, YOU CAN'T GO PAST
APPLE PIE. YOU MAY NEED TO
PRACTCE MAKING THIS PIE A FEW
TIMES BECAUSE GLUTEN-FREE
PASTRY CAN BE A BIT MORE
TRICKY TO WORK WITH THAN
PASTRY BASED ON WHEAT FLOUR.

nutrition per serving (8): Energy 258 Cal

Fat 10.1 g

Saturated fat 6.3 g

Protein 1.8 g

Carbohydrate 39.8 g

Fiber 1.7 g

Cholesterol 52 mg

APPLE AND BERRY PIE

14 oz can apple filling ^{GF}

3 tbsp sugar

1 tsp grated lemon zest

1 tbsp polenta

**1 quantity gluten-free sweet shortcrust
    pastry (Basics)**

1½ cups mixed fresh or frozen berries

raw (demerara) sugar, to sprinkle

PREP TIME: 30 MINUTES + CHILLING
COOKING TIME: 45 MINUTES
SERVINGS 6–8

Preheat the oven to 400°F. Lightly grease a pie dish that is 7 in across the base. Put the apples, caster sugar, lemon zest and polenta in a bowl and stir to combine.

Roll the pastry between two sheets of baking paper to a rough 12 in circle. Carefully turn the pastry into the prepared dish with the pastry overlapping the edge of the dish.

Stir the berries through the apple mixture, then add the apple and berry mixture to the center of the pastry. Fold over the overlapping edges leaving the fruit in the center exposed. Sprinkle the pastry with raw sugar.

Put the dish on a baking tray. Bake for 35-45 minutes, or until the pastry is crisp and lightly browned. Cover with foil if browning too much. Serve hot or warm.

HINTS:
- If you can't find a gluten-free version of canned pie apple, then use homemade stewed apples instead.
- If you have diabetes, you can replace the caster sugar with sucralose.
- Low-fat gluten-free vanilla ice cream or custard is delicious with this pie.

SPICED CREAMED RICE WITH APRICOTS

THIS CREAMY DESSERT IS BOTH DELICIOUS AND VERSATILE. YOU CAN ADD SOME CHOPPED BLANCHED ALMONDS TO THE MIXTURE IF YOU LIKE.

24 dried apricot halves

3 cups skim milk

½ cup arborio rice

1 vanilla bean, split lengthways

¼ tsp ground nutmeg

pinch of ground cardamom

¾ cup sugar

2 cinnamon sticks

2 tsp grated orange zest

3 tbsp orange juice

PREP TIME: 10 MINUTES +
  30 MINUTES SOAKING
COOKING TIME: 50 MINUTES
SERVINGS 4—6

Put the apricots in a heatproof bowl, cover with boiling water and leave to soak for 30 minutes, or until the apricots are plump.

Pour the milk into a saucepan, add the rice, vanilla bean, nutmeg and cardamom and bring to a boil. Reduce the heat and simmer gently, stirring frequently, for 25 minutes, or until the rice is soft and creamy and has absorbed most of the milk. Remove from the heat.

Remove the vanilla bean, scrape out the seeds with the tip of a knife and mix them into the rice. Stir in the caster sugar.

Meanwhile, to make the sugar syrup, put the sugar, cinnamon sticks, orange zest and juice in a saucepan with 2½ cups water. Bring to a boil, then reduce the heat and simmer for 10 minutes. Drain the apricots and add to the pan. Return to a boil, then reduce the heat to low and simmer for 5 minutes, or until soft. Remove the apricots with a slotted spoon. Return the sauce to a boil, then boil until reduced by half. Remove from the heat, cool a little and pour over the apricots. Serve the apricots with the creamed rice.

HINTS:
- If you're lactose intolerant, you can use rice milk or light gluten-free soy milk instead of the skim milk.
- If you have diabetes, you can lower the GI of this dish by replacing the arborio rice (medium GI) with a lower GI rice, such as koshikari or doongara. You can also replace the sugar with sucralose. This will reduce the calorie and carbohydrate content and help reduce the GI.

nutrition per serving (6): Energy 257 Cal; Fat 0.3 g; Saturated fat 0.2 g; Protein 6.6 g; Carbohydrate 57.9 g; Fiber 1.6 g; Cholesterol 4 mg

APPLE SNOW

THIS LIGHT REFRESHING DESSERT IS LOW GI AND LOW IN FAT AND CALORIES.
IT'S A GREAT CHOICE FOR PEOPLE WITH DIABETES OR LACTOSE INTOLERANCE
AS WELL AS THOSE WATCHING THEIR WEIGHT

4 green apples, peeled, cored and chopped
1 tsp sugar
½ tsp ground cinnamon
2 tsp powdered gelatin
3 egg whites

PREP TIME: 10 MINUTES +
30 MINUTES REFRIGERATION
COOKING TIME: 10 MINUTES
SERVINGS 4

Put the chopped apples, sugar, cinnamon and 3 tablespoons water in a saucepan. Simmer, covered, for 8 minutes, or until tender. Mash until puréed.

Sprinkle the gelatin over 1 tablespoon of water in a small heatproof bowl and leave to go spongy. Put the bowl in a saucepan of just boiled water, off the heat (the water should come halfway up the bowl). Stir to dissolve. Stir into the hot purée.

Beat the egg whites until stiff peaks form, then fold into the hot purée—the heat should slightly cook the whites. Spoon the mixture into glass bowls or parfait glasses, then refrigerate for at least 30 minutes before serving.

HINT:
- This dessert has a low GI with or without sugar. However, if you have diabetes and prefer to use sucralose instead of sugar, substitute the sugar with ½ teaspoon sucralose. This will slightly lower the carbohydrate and calorie content and will reduce your blood-sugar response.

nutrition per serving: Energy 91 Cal; Fat 0.2 g; Saturated fat 0 g; Protein 4.5 g; Carbohydrate 18.8 g; Fiber 3 g; Cholesterol 0 mg

STRAWBERRY AND RASPBERRY PARFAIT

3 oz packet diet strawberry gelatin dessert
1⅔ cups strawberries, hulled
16 oz low-fat vanilla ice cream GF
1 cup raspberries

PREP TIME: 10 MINUTES +
1 HOUR SETTING
COOKING TIME: NIL
SERVINGS 6

Put the gelatin in a heatproof bowl and pour over 1 cup boiling water. Stir to dissolve the crystals, then add 1 cup cold water. Put the bowl in the refrigerator for at least 1 hour, or until set.

Process the strawberries in a food processor for 15 seconds until blended to a pulp.

Layer the gelatin, strawberry purée and ice cream into six parfait glasses. Top with raspberries, then serve immediately.

HINTS:
- Use thawed frozen raspberries if fresh are not available.
- This dessert has a low GI and is therefore suitable for people with diabetes.
- If you are lactose intolerant, you can use a lactose-free, gluten-free vanilla dessert, such as a soy "ice cream" (available in the ice-cream section of supermarkets).

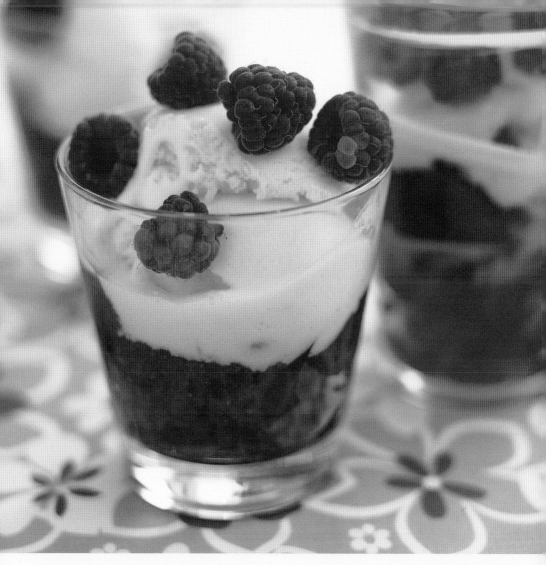

BOTH KIDS AND ADULTS WILL LOVE THIS FUN DESSERT, WHICH IS REALLY EASY TO MAKE. THE BERRIES ADD A BURST OF COLOR, FLAVOR, FIBER AND ANTIOXIDANTS.

nutrition per serving: Energy 167 Cal

Fat 2.7 g

Saturated fat 1.7 g

Protein 18.1 g

Carbohydrate 18 g

Fiber 1.8 g

Cholesterol 8 mg

137

PEACHES WITH RICOTTA CREAM

Dessert doesn't have to be a guilt-ridden indulgence: it can be an opportunity to add some more nutritious foods to your diet and reach your daily quota of fresh fruit.

4 large peaches, unpeeled
2 cups unsweetened apple juice
1 tbsp sugar
2 tsp lemon juice
3 tbsp flaked almonds, lightly toasted

Prep time: 20 minutes
Cooking time: 10 minutes
Servings 4

RICOTTA CREAM
7 oz low-fat ricotta cheese
1 tsp sugar
1 tsp natural vanilla extract
1 tsp grated lemon zest

Cut the peaches in half and remove the pit. Heat the apple juice in a saucepan over medium heat, then add the sugar and lemon juice and stir until dissolved. Add the peach halves and poach, covered, over low heat for 5–8 minutes, or until just tender when pierced with a knife. Remove with a slotted spoon and peel away the skins. Cool. Reserve the poaching juice.

To make the ricotta cream, put the ricotta, sugar, vanilla and lemon zest in a bowl and beat with electric beaters until smooth. Cover with plastic wrap, then refrigerate to firm.

Serve the peach halves with a little of the reserved juice, then spoon over the ricotta cream and sprinkle with the almonds.

HINTS:
• Use nectarines instead of the peaches, if you prefer.
• If fresh peaches are out of season, use an 28 oz canned peach halves in natural juice, drained but reserving a little of the juice for serving.
• This is a low-GI dessert but people with diabetes can use a sweetener like sucralose instead of the sugar to reduce the GI and calorie content even further.

nutrition per serving: Energy 223 Cal; Fat 7.7 g; Saturated fat 3 g; Protein 8.3 g; Carbohydrate 29.2 g; Fiber 3.5 g; Cholesterol 21 mg

PASSIONFRUIT SORBET

SORBET IS A LIGHT REFRESHING DESSERT THAT'S THE PERFECT WAY TO END A MEAL. BEING LOWER IN FAT AND CALORIES THAN ICE CREAM IT'S A MUCH HEALTHIER CHOICE, SO YOU CAN INDULGE WITHOUT GUILT.

14 oz canned peach slices in natural juice
14 oz canned pear halves in natural juice
3 tbsp sugar
4 tbsp fresh passionfruit pulp
1 tbsp lemon juice
2 egg whites
fresh fruit, to serve

PREP TIME: 15 MINUTES + FREEZING
COOKING TIME: NIL
SERVINGS 6

Drain the canned fruit and reserve the juice. Put the reserved juice and sugar in a small saucepan. Stir over low heat for 2 minutes until the sugar has dissolved. Cool.

Strain the passionfruit pulp into a small bowl, reserving the seeds. Put the strained passionfruit juice, the drained canned fruit, the cooled fruit juice and lemon juice in a food processor. Blend until smooth. Stir in the reserved passionfruit seeds.

Pour into a shallow 11 x 7 pan and freeze for 3 hours, stirring occasionally, until the mixture is icy. Use a fork to roughly mash the mixture. Put in a bowl and beat with electric beaters until smooth and creamy looking.

Beat the egg whites until firm peaks form, then fold into the creamed fruit mixture until just combined. Do not over-mix. Spoon into a 6 cup loaf pan. Cover with plastic wrap and freeze until firm.

To serve, put the tin in the refrigerator for about 15 minutes to allow the sorbet to soften a little. Use an ice-cream scoop and serve 2–3 scoops of sorbet per person. Serve with fruit.

HINTS:
- If you have diabetes, you can replace the sugar with an equal amount of sucralose, which will reduce the GI and calorie content of the dessert. Choose low-GI fruit such as passionfruit, berries or stone fruit.
- You will need 3–4 large passionfruit to yield 4 tablespoons of pulp.

nutrition per serving: Energy 76 Cal; Fat 0.05 g; Saturated fat 0 g; Protein 2.4 g; Carbohydrate 16.3 g; Fiber 4 g; Cholesterol 0 mg

139

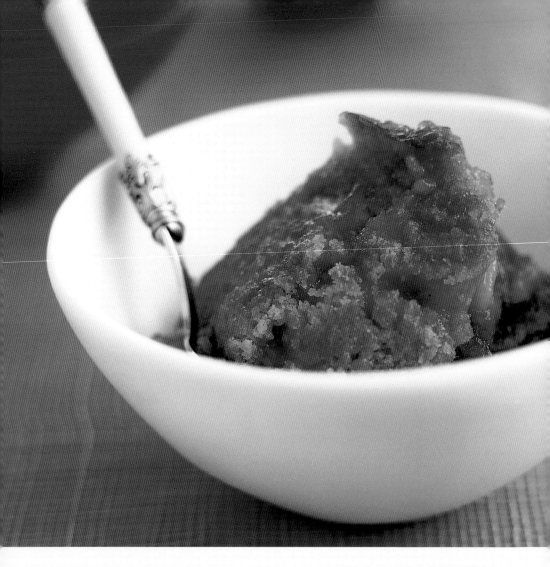

WARMING, COMFORTING PUDDINGS OFTEN TOP THE LIST OF FAVORITE WINTERTIME DESSERTS AND THIS ONE IS NO EXCEPTION.

nutrition per serving: Energy 408 Cal
Fat 11.1 g
Saturated fat 6.5 g
Protein 4.8 g
Carbohydrate 72.8 g
Fiber 1.9 g
Cholesterol 61 mg

BUTTERSCOTCH PUDDING

1¼ cups gluten-free self-rising flour

1 tsp gluten-free baking powder

⅓ cup firmly packed brown sugar

⅔ cup milk

¼ cup unsalted butter, melted, cooled

1 egg

1 tbsp golden syrup or pure maple syrup

¾ cup firmly packed brown sugar, extra

2 tbsp golden syrup or pure maple
  syrup, extra

PREP TIME: 20 MINUTES
COOKING TIME: 45 MINUTES
SERVINGS 4—6

Preheat the oven to 325°F. Lightly grease a 5-cup ovenproof dish.

Sift the flour and baking powder into a large bowl. Stir in the sugar, then make a well in the center. In a separate bowl, whisk the milk, butter, egg and golden syrup or maple syrup together. Pour into the well in the dry ingredients and whisk until a smooth batter forms. Pour into the prepared dish. Place the dish on a baking tray.

Sprinkle the extra brown sugar over the batter. Combine the extra golden syrup or maple syrup and 1⅔ cups boiling water and carefully pour over the batter. Bake the pudding for 35–45 minutes, or until a skewer inserted halfway into the pudding comes out clean.

Set the pudding aside for 5–10 minutes to allow the sauce to thicken slightly before serving.

HINT:
• To make this free of dairy and egg, replace the milk with gluten-free rice drink, the butter with dairy-free margarine and the egg with egg replacer.

CHOCOLATE SELF-SAUCING PUDDING

THIS RECIPE IS A GLUTEN-FREE VERSION OF A FAMILY FAVORITE AND IT MAKES THE PERFECT FINISHING TOUCH TO END A SPECIAL MEAL.

1¼ cups soy-containing, gluten-free, selfrising flour
1 tsp gluten-free baking powder
⅓ cup firmly packed brown sugar
½ cup milk
2 tbsp pure unsweetened cocoa powder GF
¼ cup unsalted butter, melted, cooled
1 egg, lightly beaten

¾ cup firmly packed brown sugar, extra
2 tbsp pure unsweetened cocoa powder GF, extra

PREP TIME: 20 MINUTES
COOKING TIME: 45 MINUTES
SERVINGS 4–6

Preheat the oven to 325°F. Lightly grease a 5-cup capacity ovenproof dish.

Sift the flour and baking powder into a large bowl and add the sugar; make a well in the center. In a separate bowl, whisk the milk and cocoa powder together until smooth. Set aside to cool. Add the butter and egg to the cocoa mixture and whisk to combine. Pour into the well in the flour mixture and whisk until a smooth, thick batter forms. Pour into the prepared dish. Place the dish on a baking tray.

Sprinkle the extra brown sugar over the batter. Whisk 1½ cups boiling water and the extra cocoa powder together until smooth. Carefully pour over the batter. Bake for 35–45 minutes, or until a skewer inserted halfway into the pudding comes out clean. Serve immediately.

HINTS:
• This recipe requires a gluten-free flour mixture that contains soy flour so check the ingredient list on the packet of flour. Flour with soy content behaves more like gluten flour and is necessary in some recipes.
• If you're lactose intolerant, replace the milk with ⅔ cup rice drink or gluten-free soy milk and use dairy-free margarine.
• If you prefer, you can substitute the cocoa powder with carob powder to make a carob self-saucing pudding.

nutrition per serving (6): Energy 375 Cal; Fat 10.5 g; Saturated fat 2.8 g; Protein 5.7 g; Carbohydrate 64.4 g; Fiber 2.1 g; Cholesterol 35 mg

APPLE SAGO PUDDING

SAGO IS DELICIOUS AND ADDS ANOTHER GLUTEN-FREE OPTION TO YOUR DIET. KIDS AND ADULTS WILL BOTH ENJOY THIS SWEET PUDDING, WHICH IS LIKE A MORE EXOTIC VERSION OF RICE PUDDING.

4 tbsp sugar
½ cup sago or tapioca
2¾ cupmilk
4 tbsp golden raisins
1 tsp natural vanilla extract
pinch of ground nutmeg
¼ tsp ground cinnamon
2 eggs, lightly beaten
3 small ripe apples (about 1 cup), peeled,
cored and very thinly sliced
1 tbsp brown sugar

PREP TIME: 15 MINUTES
COOKING TIME: 50 MINUTES
SERVINGS 4

Preheat the oven to 350°F. Grease a 6-cup ceramic soufflé dish. Place the sugar, sago, milk and raisins in a saucepan. Heat the mixture, stirring often. Bring to a boil, then reduce the heat and simmer for 5 minutes.

Stir in the vanilla extract, nutmeg, cinnamon, egg and the apple slices, then pour the mixture into the prepared dish. Sprinkle with the brown sugar and bake for 45 minutes, or until set and golden brown.

HINT:

- Sago is similar to tapioca and is a dried starchy granule extracted from the pith of a type of palm tree. Cooks in the South Pacific frequently use sago for baking, thickening soups and making puddings and other desserts. It's a high-carbohydrate food, but its GI value has not yet been measured.

nutrition per serving: Energy 387 Cal; Fat 8.7 g; Saturated fat 4.7 g; Protein 8.9 g; Carbohydrate 68.5 g; Fiber 2.3 g; Cholesterol 114 mg

BAKED RAISIN APPLES

4 cooking apples
⅓ cup firmly packed brown sugar
1½ tbsp chopped raisins
½ tsp ground cinnamon (optional)
2 tbsp unsalted butter
low-fat plain yogurt or ricotta cream
  (page 138), to serve

PREP TIME: 10 MINUTES
COOKING TIME: 35 MINUTES
SERVINGS 4

Preheat the oven to 425°F. Use an apple corer to remove the core of the apples, then score the skin around the middle.

Combine the sugar, raisins and cinnamon in a bowl. Place each apple on a piece of heavyduty foil and stuff it with the filling. Spread a little butter over the top of each apple, then wrap the foil securely around the apples. Bake for about 35 minutes, or until cooked. Serve with yogurt or ricotta cream.

HINTS:
- Use apples of a similar size so they all cook evenly. The apples can also be baked in a covered barbecue.
- If you choose a flavored yogurt over plain, check the ingredient list to ensure it doesn't contain any gluten.
- If you prefer, serve the apples with gluten-free ice cream.

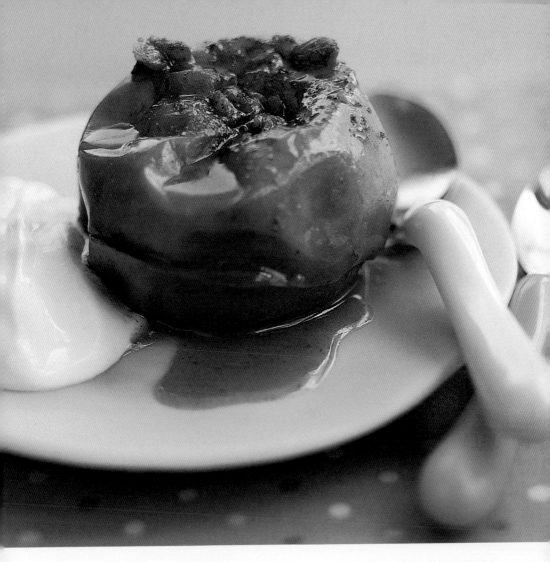

A SIMPLY DELICIOUS DESSERT
THAT PROVIDES A SWEET DOSE
OF FIBER. THE COOKED APPLE
SKIN MAY NEED TO BE REMOVED
BEFORE BEING SERVED TO VERY
YOUNG CHILDREN.

nutrition per serving: Energy 205 Cal
Fat 4.4 g
Saturated fat 2.7 g
Protein 0.7 g
Carbohydrate 40.8 g
Fiber 3.5 g
Cholesterol 13 mg

CREPES WITH COFFEE SAUCE

YOU CAN TEAM THESE CREPES WITH A NUMBER OF DIFFERENT TOPPINGS, SUCH AS PURE FRUIT JAM, LEMON JUICE AND SUGAR, OR EVEN GLUTEN-FREE CHOCOLATE SPREAD.

COFFEE SAUCE
2 tbsp golden syrup or pure maple syrup
3 tsp instant coffee powder
2 tbsp pure maize cornstarch GF
1 cup firmly packed brown sugar

CREPES
1¼ cups gluten-free all-purpose flour
2 tsp gluten-free baking powder
1 egg
2 tbsp canola oil

PREP TIME: 35 MINUTES
COOKING TIME: 25 MINUTES
MAKES 10

To make the coffee sauce, combine the syrup, coffee powder, cornstarch and sugar in a frying pan. Add 1 cup water and blend. Put the pan over medium heat. Stir constantly until the mixture boils and thickens. Reduce the heat and simmer for 2–3 minutes. Set aside.

To make the crepes, sift the flour and baking powder into a bowl. Gradually add the combined egg, 1 tablespoon of the oil and 1¼ cups water, stirring well until the batter is smooth and the consistency of thin cream, adding more water if needed. Strain into a vessel with a pouring lip.

Lightly brush an 8 in frying pan with a little of the remaining oil and heat over medium heat. Pour in just enough crepe batter to thinly cover the bottom of the pan. When the top of the crepe starts to set, turn it over with a spatula. After browning the second side, transfer to a plate. Repeat with the remaining crepe batter, greasing the pan between each. Fold each crepe in four to form a triangle.

Reheat the sauce in a frying pan over low heat. Put the crepes in the pan and heat gently until warmed through. Place the crepes on two serving plates and spoon any extra warm sauce over the top.

HINT:
• If you have diabetes, use pure maple syrup (low GI) instead of golden syrup (medium GI).

nutrition per crepe with sauce: Energy 223 Cal; Fat 4.3 g; Saturated fat 0.4 g; Protein 1.1 g; Carbohydrate 45.7 g; Fiber 0.4 g; Cholesterol 19 mg

POACHED PEARS IN VANILLA–LEMON SYRUP

THESE PEARS ARE DELICIOUS EITHER WARM OR COLD AND MAKE A STYLISH, YET HEALTHY, DESSERT—GOOD ENOUGH TO SERVE AT DINNER PARTIES.

¾ cup sugar

1 vanilla bean, split lengthways and scraped

1 strip lemon zest

1½ tsp lemon grass tea leaves

4 large firm pears, peeled with stems intact

4 tbsp low-fat plain yogurt

PREP TIME: 15 MINUTES
COOKING TIME: 50 MINUTES
SERVINGS 4

Put the sugar, vanilla bean and lemon zest in a large saucepan with 2 cups water. Put the lemon grass in a tea-infuser ball or small muslin (cheesecloth) bag, and add to the saucepan. Heat over low heat, stirring occasionally, until the sugar melts.

Bring to a boil, then reduce to a simmer and add the pears, laying them on their sides. Cover and simmer, turning occasionally, for 30 minutes, or until the pears are tender when pierced with a skewer.

Remove the pears with a slotted spoon and set aside to cool. Meanwhile, increase the heat to high and simmer the syrup for 8–10 minutes, or until reduced by half and thickened slightly. Remove the vanilla bean, lemon zest and lemon grass tea. Serve the pears drizzled with the syrup and a dollop of the yogurt on the side.

HINTS:
- If you have diabetes, you can make this a low-GI dessert by using sucralose instead of sugar. This will also reduce the calorie content.
- If you place the lemon grass tea in a tea-infuser ball or muslin bag, it can readily be removed, as it is too fine to be strained from the syrup.
- You can use a flavored yogurt instead of plain, if you prefer; remember to check the label because many flavored yogurts contain gluten.

nutrition per serving: Energy 293 Cal; Fat 0.2 g; Saturated fat 0.02 g; Protein 1.8 g; Carbohydrate 72 g; Fiber 3.7 g; Cholesterol 1 mg

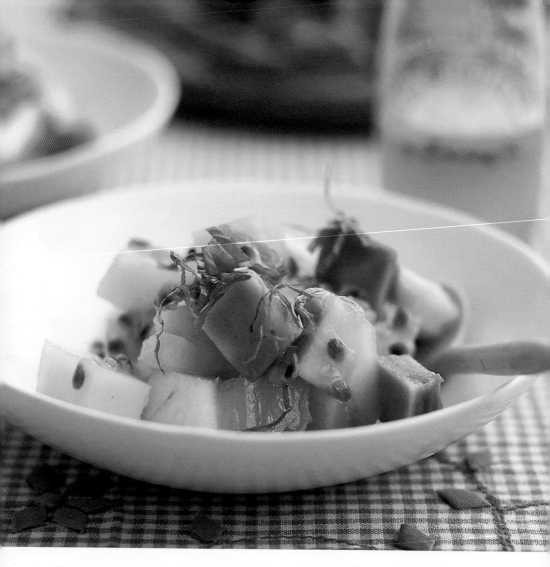

THIS REFRESHING BLEND OF
TROPICAL FRUIT IS A GOOD
SOURCE OF FIBER, VITAMIN C,
POTASSIUM AND OTHER
ANTIOXIDANTS AND MAKES A
HEALTHY, GUILT-FREE DESSERT.

nutrition per serving: Energy 224 Cal

Fat 0.8 g

Saturated fat 0.01 g

Protein 3.4 g

Carbohydrate 47.8 g

Fiber 7.2 g

Cholesterol 0 g

LEMON GRASS AND GINGER FRUIT SALAD

3 tbsp sugar
about ¾ in piece of fresh ginger, thinly
    sliced
1 lemon grass stem, bruised and halved
pulp from 1 large passionfruit
1 papaya
½ honeydew melon
1 large mango

1 small pineapple
12 lychees
1 large handful mint, shredded, to serve

PREP TIME: 20 MINUTES
COOKING TIME: 10 MINUTES
SERVINGS 4

Place the sugar, ginger and lemon grass in a small saucepan, add ½ cup water and stir over low heat to dissolve the sugar. Boil for 5 minutes, or until reduced to 4 tablespoons, then set aside to cool. Strain the syrup and add the passionfruit pulp.

Peel and seed the papaya and melon. Cut the papaya and the melon into 1½ in cubes. Peel the mango and cut the flesh into cubes, discarding the pit. Peel, halve and core the pineapple and cut into cubes. Peel the lychees, then make a slit in the flesh and remove the seed.

Place all the fruit in a large serving bowl. Pour the syrup over the fruit, or serve separately, if you prefer. Garnish with the mint.

HINT:
• Serve with gluten-free low-fat yogurt for a calcium boost.

BAKING

WALNUT AND SEED BREAD

3 eggs, lightly beaten

3 tbsp canola or olive oil

4 cups soy-containing, gluten-free all
purpose flour

1 tsp brown sugar

2 tsp dried yeast GF

½ tsp salt

¼ tsp tartaric acid

1 tbsp each of sunflower seeds, pepitas
and poppy seeds

⅔ cup chopped walnuts

canola or olive oil, extra, for glazing

mixed seeds, to sprinkle

PREP TIME: 30 MINUTES +
50 MINUTES RISING
COOKING TIME: 45 MINUTES
SERVINGS: 8–10

Preheat the oven to 400°F. Lightly grease a 9 in round cake tin and line the base with baking paper.

Beat together the eggs, oil and 2 cups warm water in a bowl. Put the flour, sugar, yeast, salt and tartaric acid in a separate large bowl. Using electric beaters, beat on a low speed for 20 seconds to combine.With the motor running, gradually beat in the egg mixture until smooth. Continue to beat for 5 minutes. Add the seeds and chopped walnuts and beat until incorporated.

Pour the batter into the prepared tin. Cover with greased plastic wrap and set aside in a warm place for 50 minutes until the batter has nearly risen to the top of the pan. Brush the top of the loaf lightly with oil and sprinkle evenly with the extra seeds. Bake for 45 minutes, or until golden brown.

Cool in the pan for 10 minutes, then turn out onto a wire rack to cool completely. Cut into slices to serve.

HINTS:

- When making this bread it's important to use a gluten-free flour mixture that includes soy flour in its composition. Soy flour acts more like gluten flour and gives a better result for the bread.
- Gluten-free yeast should be stored in the freezer.
- Gluten-free breads can sink after being taken out of the oven if the kitchen is too humid or if the bread was left to rise too long before being placed in the oven. If you make a yeast-leavened dough that doesn't rise properly, make it again and add 1 teaspoon of vinegar or a pinch of citric acid to the water before you add the yeast.
- Store the bread in an airtight container in the refrigerator for up to 5 days.

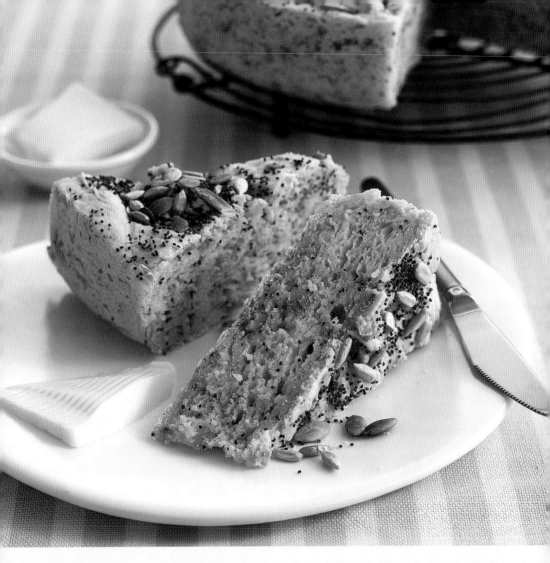

MANY PEOPLE FIND THEY MISS WHOLEGRAIN BREAD AFTER THEY START A GLUTEN-FREE DIET. THIS RECIPE GIVES YOU A GLUTEN-FREE BREAD THAT HAS SOME TEXTURE AND BITE TO IT. THE SEEDS AND NUTS ADD FIBER AND MINERALS.

nutrition per slice (10): Energy 284 Ca)
Fat 14.8 g
Saturated fat 1.7 g
Protein 4.4 g
Carbohydrate 33.1 g
Fiber 2 g
Cholesterol 56 mg

153

WHITE BREAD

ENJOY THE SMELL OF BREAD BAKING IN THE OVEN AND MAKE THIS
GLUTENFREE VERSION OF WHITE BREAD. YOU CAN ADD MORE FIBER TO THIS
LOAF BY ADDING RICE BRAN TO THE DRY INGREDIENTS.

2 cups milk

4 tsp dried yeast GF

1 tbsp sugar

3⅔ cups gluten-free all-purpose flour

2 tsp salt

4 tbsp canola or olive oil

1 egg

2 tbsp roasted buckwheat kernels (groats)
   (optional)

2 tbsp canola or olive oil, extra, for glazing

PREP TIME: 40 MINUTES

COOKING TIME: 55 MINUTES

SERVINGS: 8—10

Preheat the oven to 425°F. Lightly grease an 8 x 4 in loaf pan.

Pour the milk into a saucepan over medium heat, bring almost to a boil, then remove from the heat and allow to cool until it is lukewarm.

Combine the yeast, sugar and the warm milk in a bowl, then stir to dissolve the yeast. Stand the bowl in a warm place for about 10 minutes, or until the mixture is frothy.

Sift the flour into a large bowl and add the salt. Make a well in the center and add the yeast mixture, oil and egg. Beat well with a wooden spoon. Pour into the prepared tin and sprinkle with buckwheat, if using. Cover loosely and place in a warm place for about 20 minutes, or until the mixture comes to the top of the pan.

Bake for 20 minutes, then reduce the heat to 400°F and bake for a further 30–35 minutes, or until cooked. Brush with the extra oil during cooking at least twice to help promote browning.

HINTS:
• Store gluten-free yeast in the freezer.
• Use a commercial gluten-free bread mixture or flour mixture that's suitable for breadmaking rather than one type of gluten-free flour—the result will be much better.
• To add more fiber to this loaf, add ½ cup rice bran with the flour.
• homemade bread is best eaten on the day of baking; alternatively, you can slice it, then freeze until required.

nutrition per slice (10): Energy 357 Cal; Fat 13.8 g; Saturated fat 2.6 g; Protein 3.5 g; Carbohydrate 53.6 g; Fiber 1.2 g; Cholesterol 25 mg

SAVORY FLAT BREAD

THIS BREAD IS GREAT FOR CHILDREN AND TEENAGERS WHO NEED A GLUTENFREE DIET AS IT MAKES A GOOD GLUTEN-FREE ALTERNATIVE TO CRACKERS AND PITA BREAD—PERFECT FOR SNACKS OR SCHOOL LUNCH BOXES.

½ cup brown rice flour
½ cup arrowroot
¾ tsp baking soda
1½ tsp cream of tartar
1 cup rice bran
1 cup chicken stock ᴳᶠ (Basics) or water
3 tbsp canola or olive oil
canola or olive oil, extra, for glazing

1 tbsp salt
1 tbsp poppy seeds

PREP TIME: 20 MINUTES
COOKING TIME: 40 MINUTES
MAKES 6—8 ROUNDS

Preheat the oven to 375°F. Grease two baking trays.

Sift the flour, arrowroot, baking soda and cream of tartar into a large bowl. Add the rice bran. Make a well in the center, then add the combined stock and oil. Beat until smooth with a wooden spoon.

Spoon heaped tablespoons of the dough onto the prepared trays.

Bake for 20 minutes. Remove from the oven, brush with oil and sprinkle with salt and poppy seeds. Return to the oven and bake for a further 15–20 minutes.

HINTS:
• Many commercial stocks contain gluten so check the label.
• The bread can be topped or split and filled. It does not freeze well but can be kept in the refrigerator for 2–3 days.

nutrition per round (8): Energy 193 Cal; Fat 11.5 g; Saturated fat 1.4 g; Protein 3.2 g; Carbohydrate 17.2 g; Fiber 4 g; Cholesterol 1 mg

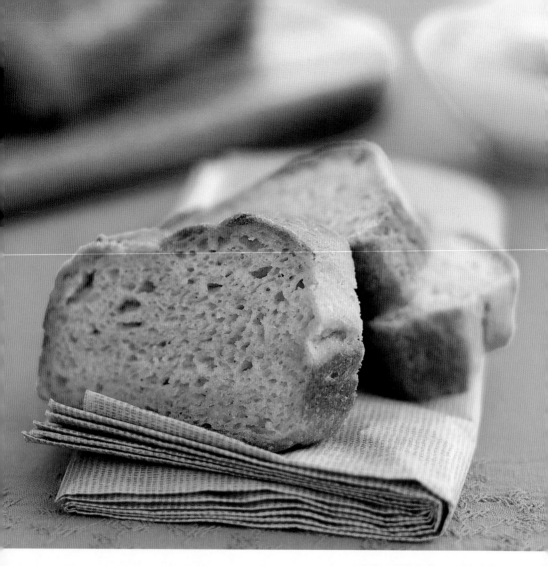

If your local shops don't sell gluten-free bread rolls, then why not make your own? Make a double batch and freeze them until needed.

nutrition per roll: Energy 311 Cal
Fat 10.4 g
Saturated fat 4.6 g
Protein 3.1 g
Carbohydrate 48.8 g
Fiber 3.3 g
Cholesterol 19 mg

BREAD ROLLS

4 tsp dried yeast ^{GF}

1 tbsp brown sugar

2 tsp guar gum or xanthan gum

2 cups gluten-free all-purpose flour

¾ cup rice flour

2 tsp salt

½ cup rice bran

¼ cup butter, melted, cooled

2 tbsp poppy seeds or sesame seeds (optional)

canola or olive oil, for brushing

PREP TIME: 40 MINUTES + RISING TIME

COOKING TIME: 35 MINUTES

MAKES 8

Preheat the oven to 400°F. Lightly grease eight 4 x 2¼ in individual loaf tins.

Combine the yeast, sugar and 2 cups warm water in a bowl, then stir to dissolve the yeast. Stand the bowl in a warm place for about 10 minutes, or until the mixture is frothy.

Sift the gum and flours into a large bowl. Add the salt and rice bran. Make a well in the center and add the yeast mixture and cooled butter. Mix well to form a soft dough. Divide into eight equal portions, then gently shape with gluten-free floured hands into an oval shape. Place in the prepared pans. Sprinkle with poppy seeds or sesame seeds, if using.

Cover loosely and place in a warm place for 45–60 minutes, or until the mixture comes to the top of the pans.

Bake for 25–30 minutes, or until cooked through. Brush with oil during cooking at least twice to help promote browning. Remove from the pans and leave to cool on a wire rack.

HINTS:
- Store gluten-free yeast in the freezer.
- Guar gum and xanthan gum are available from health-food stores and some local celiac organizations. These are useful products because they mimic the properties of gluten and help reduce crumbling in baked goods.
- The bread rolls are best eaten on the day they are made, but they can be frozen for up to 2 months.

CHEESE PINWHEELS

THESE GLUTEN-FREE PINWHEELS ARE A GOOD ALTERNATIVE TO SAVORY SCROLLS AND WILL HELP SATISFY A CRAVING FOR SOMETHING CHEESY OR SAVORY. THEY ARE A GOOD ADDITION TO LUNCH BOXES OR PICNIC HAMPERS.

¾ cup potato flour
1 cup rice flour
2 tsp gluten-free baking powder
⅓ cup butter
3–4 tbsp milk
milk or water, for glazing
1 tbsp poppy seeds

RICOTTA FILLING
¾ cup ricotta cheese
2 spring onions (scallions), finely chopped

PREP TIME: 20 MINUTES
COOKING TIME: 15 MINUTES
SERVINGS: 4–6

Preheat the oven to 350°F. Lightly grease an 8 in square pan.

Sift the dry ingredients into a bowl. Rub the butter in with your fingertips until the mixture resembles fine breadcrumbs. Make a well in the center. Add enough milk to make a soft dough. Turn out onto a rice-floured board and knead lightly.

Roll the dough into a ¼ in thick rectangle between two sheets of baking paper. Turn and release the paper frequently to prevent the dough from sticking to the paper.

To make the ricotta filling, beat the ricotta cheese in a bowl until creamy. Add the spring onions and mix well. Spread the filling over the dough.

Use the baking paper to help you roll up the dough. Once you have a roll, cut it into ¾ in thick slices. Place the slices, cut side up, into the prepared pan. Glaze with milk or water and sprinkle the top with poppy seeds. Bake for 12–15 minutes. Serve hot or cold.

nutrition per serving (6): Energy 350 Cal; Fat 17 g; Saturated fat 10.5 g; Protein 7.4 g; Carbohydrate 40.1 g; Fiber 2.4 g; Cholesterol 53 mg

SCONES

JUST BECAUSE YOU FOLLOW A GLUTEN-FREE DIET DOESN'T MEAN YOU CAN'T ENJOY A TRADITIONAL AFTERNOON TEA. THIS RECIPE GIVES YOU A GLUTENFREE VERSION OF SCONES. SERVE WITH JAM AND CREAM, HOT OR COLD.

3⅔ cups gluten-free self-rising flour
3 tsp gluten-free baking powder
⅓ cup butter, softened
1 tbsp sugar
1¼ cups milk
whipped cream, to serve
strawberry jam ᴳᶠ **(Basics), to serve**

PREP TIME: 10 MINUTES
COOKING TIME: 15 MINUTES
MAKES 12

Preheat the oven to 425°F. Line a baking tray with a sheet of baking paper.

Sift the flour, baking powder and a pinch of salt into a large bowl. Use your fingertips to rub the butter into the flour until it resembles fine breadcrumbs. Stir in the sugar. Add the milk and use a round-bladed knife to mix until the dough just comes together.

Turn out onto a surface lightly dusted with gluten-free flour and knead until combined. Press or roll out until the dough is about ¾ in thick. Use a 2¼ in round cutter to cut out the dough. Place on the lined tray about ½ in apart. Re-roll and cut any remaining dough.

Bake for 12–15 minutes, or until cooked. Serve warm with whipped cream and strawberry jam.

HINTS:
• Look for a gluten-free flour mixture that is suitable for baked goods. You will get a better result than by using a gluten-free flour made up of only one type of flour.
• If you're lactose intolerant, replace the milk with rice drink or soy milk and make sure to buy a gluten-free flour mixture that doesn't contain milk powder.
• If you're invited to an afternoon tea at a friend's house, take a container of these scones with you, so you have something suitable to eat.

nutrition per scone: Energy 239 Cal; Fat 6.8 g; Saturated fat 4.3 g; Protein 1.6 g; Carbohydrate 42.7 g; Fiber 4.8 g; Cholesterol 20 mg

SAVORY CORN AND CHIVE MUFFINS

2 cups gluten-free self-rising flour
2 tsp gluten-free baking powder
2 tbsp brown sugar
½ cup drained, canned corn kernels
2 tbsp finely chopped fresh chives
1 cup milk
4 tbsp canola or olive oil
2 eggs, lightly beaten

PREP TIME: 15 MINUTES
COOKING TIME: 20 MINUTES
MAKES 10

Preheat the oven to 350°F. Lightly grease a regular muffin tin.

Sift the flour and baking powder into a large bowl. Stir in the sugar, corn and chives, then make a well in the center. In a separate bowl, combine the milk, oil and eggs. Pour into the well in the dry ingredients. Use a large metal spoon to mix until just combined. Divide the batter evenly among ten of the prepared muffin holes.

Bake for 18–20 minutes, or until a skewer inserted in the center comes out clean. Leave in the tray for 5 minutes before turning out onto a wire rack to cool.

HINTS:
- A combination of gluten-free flours usually produces a better product than using only one type of flour. This is why many commercial gluten-free flour mixtures contain a number of different flours.
- If you're lactose intolerant, replace the milk with rice drink or gluten-free soy milk.
- Like many gluten-free baked goods, these muffins don't stay fresh for very long. They need to be eaten on the day they are made or they can be frozen for up to 1 month.

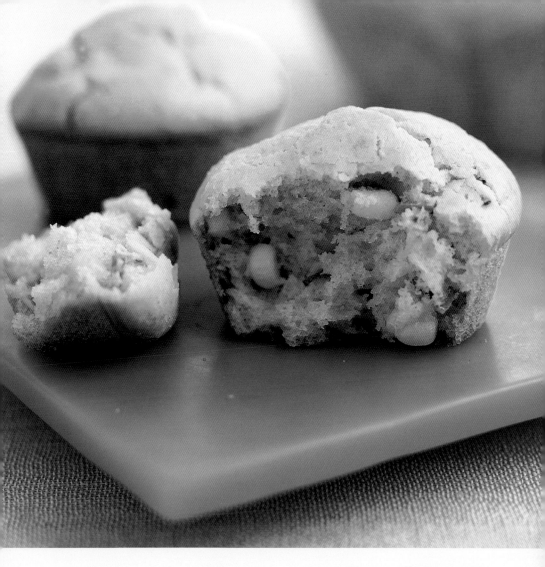

IT'S OFTEN HARD TO FIND GLUTENFREE
FOOD WHEN YOU'RE ON THE
MOVE, SO BE PREPARED TO EAT
WELL BY TAKING SUITABLE FOODS
WITH YOU. THESE LITTLE MUFFINS
ARE PERFECT BECAUSE THEY ARE
LIGHT AND PORTABLE.

nutrition per muffin: Energy 226 Cal

Fat 10 g

Saturated fat 1.5 g

Protein 3.9 g

Carbohydrate 29.4 g

Fiber 3.8 g

Cholesterol 41 mg

PIKELETS

PIKELETS MAKE A GREAT AFTERNOON TEA AT THE END OF A SCHOOL DAY OR ON A LAZY WEEKEND. HUNGRY KIDS AND TEENAGERS WILL REALLY APPRECIATE THEM.

¾ cup gluten-free all-purpose flour
½ tsp baking soda
1 tsp cream of tartar
4 tbsp rice bran
2 eggs, separated
1 tbsp canola oil
strawberry jam GF (Basics), to serve

PREP TIME: 15 MINUTES
COOKING TIME: 25 MINUTES
MAKES ABOUT 24

Sift the flour, baking soda and cream of tartar into a bowl. Mix in the rice bran. Make a well in the center. In a separate bowl, combine the egg yolks, oil and 1 cup water. Add to the well in the dry ingredients. Beat well until smooth.

Beat the egg whites in the small bowl of an electric mixer until stiff peaks form, then fold into the batter using a large spoon.

Spray a non-stick frying pan lightly with canola or olive oil and place over medium heat. Place tablespoonfuls of the mixture in the pan, allowing room for spreading.When the mixture starts to set and bubbles burst, turn over and brown the other side. Place on a wire rack to cool. Repeat with the remaining mixture. Serve the warm pikelets topped with strawberry jam.

HINTS:
• Pikelets are a popular Australian snack, best described as a mini pancake, sort of like a blini.
• Pikelets can be frozen.When ready to eat, thaw them, then reheat briefly in a warm oven.
• Experiment with different toppings for the pikelets, such as maple syrup, honey, pure fruit jam or your favourite spread.

nutrition per pikelet: Energy 36 Cal; Fat 1.5 g; Saturated fat 0.2 g; Protein 0.8 g; Carbohydrate 4.6 g; Fiber 0.4 g; Cholesterol 16 mg

JAM COOKIES

BE PREPARED TO COOK LOTS OF THESE—YOU MIGHT NOT BE ABLE TO MAKE THESE COOKIES FAST ENOUGH TO KEEP UP WITH THE DEMAND.

½ cup unsalted butter
½ cup sugar
¾ cup rice flour
¼ tsp gluten-free baking powder
½ cup strawberry jam GF (Basics)

PREP TIME: 20 MINUTES
COOKING TIME: 15 MINUTES
MAKES ABOUT 24

Preheat the oven to 375°F. Lightly grease two baking trays.

Use electric beaters to beat the butter and sugar until light and fluffy. Sift in the flour and baking powder, then stir together. Add 1 tablespoon water and stir until well blended and a dough forms.

Shape the dough into walnut-sized balls, then space them out on the prepared baking trays—you should have about 24 balls.

Make an indentation in each cookie using the handle of a wooden spoon. Put ¼ teaspoon jam in each cookie. Bake for 10–15 minutes, or until light golden. Cool on wire racks.

HINTS:
• You may find the dough easier to work with if you refrigerate it for 30 minutes before rolling the dough into balls.
• The dough can be made ahead of time and stored, covered, in the refrigerator for 2–3 days before baking.
• For a special treat, you can add ½ cup gluten-free chocolate chips to the dough mixture for jam and chocolate chip cookies.

nutrition per cookie: Energy 74 Cal; Fat 3.2 g; Saturated fat 2 g; Protein 0.4 g; Carbohydrate 11.2 g; Fiber 0.2 g; Cholesterol 10 mg

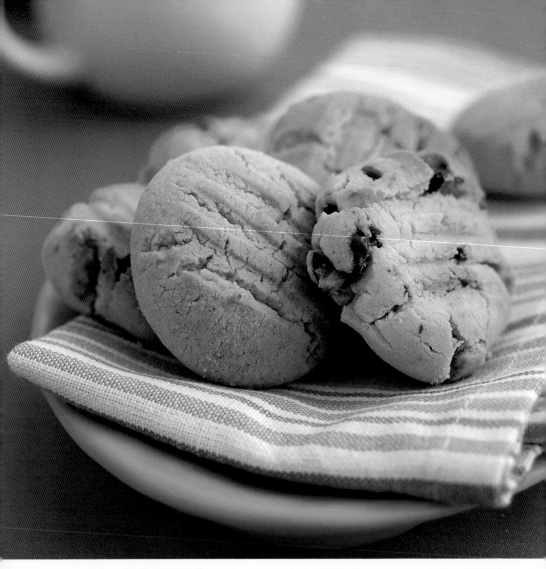

ONCE YOU'VE COOKED THESE
COOKIES A FEW TIMES YOU MAY
WANT TO START EXPERIMENTING
BY ADDING NUTS, CHOCOLATE,
CAROB OR EVEN DRIED FRUIT TO
THE BASIC MIXTURE.

nutrition per cookie: Energy 111 Cal
Fat 5.9 g
Saturated fat 3.8 g
Protein 0.5 g
Carbohydrate 13.8 g
Fiber 0.4 g
Cholesterol 18 mg

VANILLA COOKIES

½ cup unsalted butter
4 tbsp sugar
1 tsp natural vanilla extract
1 cup gluten-free all-purpose flour
½ cup gluten-free self-rising flour

PREP TIME: 15 MINUTES
COOKING TIME: 15 MINUTES
MAKES ABOUT 18

Preheat the oven to 325°F. Line two baking trays with baking paper.

Beat the butter, sugar and vanilla extract in the small bowl of an electric mixer for 1–2 minutes, or until well combined. Sift the flours into the butter mixture. Use a wooden spoon to mix until well combined. Use your hands to shape the mixture into a soft dough.

Shape tablespoons of the mixture into balls and place on the prepared trays. Use a fork to flatten the balls until about ⅜ in thick. Bake for 12–15 minutes, swapping the trays around once, until light golden. Transfer the cookies to a wire rack to cool.

HINTS:
- Make sure you store gluten-free flours separately from gluten-containing flours, in labelled containers, to avoid cross-contamination. Brown rice flour and soy flour should be stored in the refrigerator, whereas other gluten-free flours can be stored in a cool dark place. For long-term storage, keep gluten-free flours in the freezer in well-sealed containers. The flour doesn't need to be thawed before being used.
- You may find the dough easier to work with if you refrigerate it for 30 minutes before shaping the dough into balls.
- If you like, you can add 3½ oz chopped gluten-free chocolate, carob, nuts or dried fruit to the dough before mixing it together with a wooden spoon.

APPLE SLICE

THIS SLICE IS DELICIOUS FOR MORNING OR AFTERNOON TEA. MAKE SURE YOU USE PURE GLUTEN-FREE CONFECTIONERS' SUGAR TO DUST THE SLICE. SOFT CONFECTIONERS' SUGAR AND CONFECTIONERS' SUGAR MIXTURES MAY CONTAIN GLUTEN.

1½ cups gluten-free self-rising flour
½ tsp gluten-free baking powder
¾ cup sugar
2 eggs, lightly beaten
3 tbsp apple juice
3 tbsp canola oil
1½cups unsweetened apples
pure confectioners' sugar GF, to serve

PREP TIME: 15 MINUTES
COOKING TIME: 35 MINUTES
MAKES ABOUT 20 PIECES

Preheat the oven to 375°F. Lightly grease an 11 x 7 in baking pan and cover the base and two long sides with baking paper.

Sift the flour and baking powder into a bowl and add the sugar. Make a well in the center. Combine the eggs, juice, oil and ½ cup cold water in a separate bowl, then add to the dry ingredients. Mix until thoroughly combined.

Spread half the batter into the prepared pan. Spread the apple sauce carefully over the top, then spoon the remaining batter gently over the apple so that it is completely covered.

Bake for 30–35 minutes, or until golden. Cool slightly in the tin, then place on a wire rack to cool completely. Dust with confectioners' sugar and cut into 20 pieces before serving.

HINTS:
- Check that you are using pure confectioners' sugar; some confectioners' sugar mixtures contain gluten.
- You can make a pear version of this slice by replacing the apple with 4 canned pear halves that have been mashed, and replacing the apple juice with pear juice.

nutrition per serving: Energy 113 Cal; Fat 3.6 g; Saturated fat 0.4 g; Protein 1.6 g; Carbohydrate 18.3 g; Fiber 0.9 g; Cholesterol 19 mg

RHUBARB MUFFINS

WITH GLUTEN-FREE FLOURS READILY AVAILABLE IN SUPERMARKETS, IT'S EASY TO MAKE YOUR OWN HOMEMADE MUFFINS. MAKE A BATCH AND FREEZE THEM SO YOU HAVE A READY SUPPLY OF GLUTEN-FREE SNACKS.

2 cups gluten-free self-rising flour
2 tsp gluten-free baking powder
¾ cup brown sugar
¾ cup milk
4 tbsp canola oil
2 eggs, lightly beaten
**½ bunch (about 7 oz) trimmed rhubarb,
  washed and cut into ¾ in pieces**

PREP TIME: 15 MINUTES
COOKING TIME: 20 MINUTES
MAKES 12

Preheat the oven to 350°F. Lightly grease a regular muffin pan.

Sift the flour and baking powder into a large bowl. Stir in the sugar and make a well in the center. In a separate bowl, combine the milk, oil and eggs. Pour into the well in the dry ingredients along with the rhubarb. Use a large spoon to mix until just combined. Divide the batter evenly among the prepared muffin cups.

Bake for 18–20 minutes, or until a skewer inserted in the center comes out clean. Leave to cool in the pan for 5 minutes before turning out onto a wire rack to cool completely.

HINTS:
- These muffins are best eaten on the day they are made but they can be frozen for up to 1 month.
- If you are lactose intolerant replace the milk with rice drink or gluten-free soy milk.

nutrition per muffin: Energy 216 Cal; Fat 8.4 g; Saturated fat 1.2 g; Protein 3.8 g; Carbohydrate 30.2 g; Fiber 1.8 g; Cholesterol 33 mg

MIXED BERRY MUFFINS

2 cups gluten-free all-purpose flour
1 tbsp gluten-free baking powder
1.2 cup baby rice cereal or rice porridge
⅔ cup sugar
2 eggs, lightly beaten
1½ cups reduced-fat milk
2 tbsp canola oil
1⅔ cups fresh or frozen mixed berries

PREP TIME: 15 MINUTES
COOKING TIME: 20 MINUTES
MAKES 12

Preheat oven to 400°F. Lightly grease 12 holes of a regular muffin pan.

Sift the flour and baking powder into a large bowl. Stir in the rice cereal and sugar and make a well in the center. In a separate bowl combine the beaten eggs, milk and oil. Pour the mixture into the well in the dry ingredients and stir briefly until the batter is just incorporated. Quickly and lightly stir through the berries. Do not over-mix. Divide the batter evenly among the prepared muffin cups.

Bake for 20 minutes, or until golden brown and risen. Leave in the pan for 5 minutes before turning out onto a wire rack to cool completely.

HINTS:
- Use dried fruit such as chopped dates, sultanas, raisins or apricots instead of the berries, if you prefer.
- If you are making these muffins for someone with diabetes, you can lower the muffins' GI by using sucralose instead of sugar. Similarly, if making these muffins for someone with lactose intolerance, use gluten-free soy milk or rice milk instead of cow's milk.

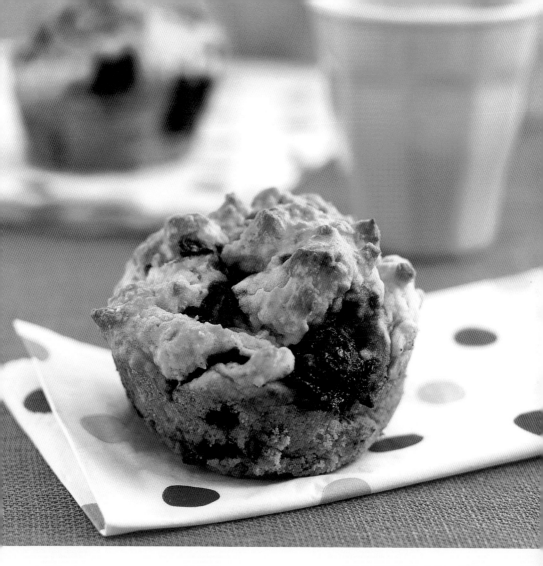

IF YOU HAVE YOUNG CHILDREN WHO NEED A GLUTEN-FREE DIET, YOU CAN MAKE BITE-SIZED MUFFINS USING A MINI MUFFIN PAN. THAT WAY, YOU'LL WASTE LESS IF YOUR CHILD CAN'T EAT A WHOLE REGULAR-SIZED MUFFIN.

nutrition per muffin: Energy 211 Cal

Fat 4.6 g

Saturated fat 0.8 g

Protein 3.3 g

Carbohydrate 38.8 g

Fiber 0.9 g

Cholesterol 34 mg

COFFEE MOUSSE MERINGUE ROLL

THIS IS SIMILAR TO A SWISS (JELLY) ROLL USING MERINGUE INSTEAD OF CAKE. THE SOPHISTICATED COFFEE MOUSSE MAKES A DELICIOUS FILLING.

COFFEE MOUSSE

4 egg yolks

3 tbsp sugar

3 tsp pure maize cornstarch GF

1½ tsp instant coffee powder

pure maize cornstarch GF**, for dusting**

4 egg whites

½ cup sugar

2 tsp pure maize cornstarch GF

pure confectioners' sugar GF**, for dusting**

PREP TIME: 35 MINUTES

COOKING TIME: 15 MINUTES

SERVINGS: 4—6

To make the coffee mousse, beat the egg yolks and sugar in the small bowl of an electric mixer until thick and creamy. In a separate small bowl, blend the cornstarch, coffee powder and ¾ cup water. Add to the egg mixture. Transfer to a saucepan and stir over low heat until the mixture boils and thickens. Pour the mixture into a bowl. Cover with plastic wrap and chill well before using.

Preheat the oven to 400°F. Lightly grease a 10 x 12 in Swiss jelly roll tin, line with baking paper, grease again and dust with cornstarch.

Beat the egg whites until light and fluffy. Gradually beat in the sugar and continue beating until the meringue is stiff and glossy. Gently fold in the cornstarch. Spread the meringue mixture evenly into the prepared pan, using a spatula.

Bake for 12–15 minutes, or until the meringue has risen and is golden brown. Quickly turn out onto a sheet of baking paper that has been coated with sifted pure confectioners' sugar. Allow to cool until lukewarm.

Spread the mousse over the meringue. Roll up from the short side using the baking paper as a guide. Place on a chilled platter. Refrigerate the roll until ready to serve, then slice.

HINT:
• If you have diabetes, you can use sucralose instead of sugar to lower the GI.

nutrition per serving: Energy 158 Cal; Fat 3.2 g; Saturated fat 1 g; Protein 4.1 g; Carbohydrate 29.3 g; Fiber 0.1 g; Cholesterol 119 mg

PUMPKIN AND COCONUT TART

THIS TART IS GREAT TO SHARE WITH FRIENDS FOR MORNING OR AFTERNOON TEA, OR YOU COULD EVEN SERVE IT FOR DESSERT WITH SOME ICE CREAM.

1 quantity gluten-free sweet shortcrust pastry (Basics)
1½ cups cooked mashed butternut squash
3 eggs, lightly beaten
¾ cup firmly packed brown sugar
½ cup sour cream
½ cup flaked coconut
3 tbsp golden syrup or pure maple syrup
pure confectioners' sugar GF, to dust

PREP TIME: 25 MINUTES
COOKING TIME: 1 ¼ HOURS
SERVINGS: 8—10

Preheat the oven to 400°F. Lightly grease a 9 in springform pan.

Roll out the pastry between two sheets of baking paper until large enough to line the prepared pan. Reserve any leftover dough.

Place the pan on a baking tray. Cover the pastry with a sheet of crumpled baking paper and fill with baking beads or rice. Bake for 10 minutes. Remove the beads and paper and bake for a further 10–15 minutes, or until lightly browned. Fill any cracks with small amounts of reserved pastry. Bake for a further 2 minutes to set. Remove from the oven and cool completely. Reduce the oven temperature to 350°F.

To make the filling, combine all the ingredients (except the confectioners' sugar) in a large bowl and mix together well. Place the cooled pastry case on a baking tray and pour in the filling.

Bake for 45 minutes; or until the filling is just set. Cool completely before serving. Dust the edges lightly with confectioners' sugar.

HINT:
• Make sure you use pure confectioners' sugar to dust the tart. Some mixtures can contain cornstarch with wheat starch in it.

nutrition per serving (10): Energy 322 Cal; Fat 14.7 g; Saturated fat 9.1 g; Protein 4.1 g; Carbohydrate 44.1 g; Fiber 1 g; Cholesterol 112 mg

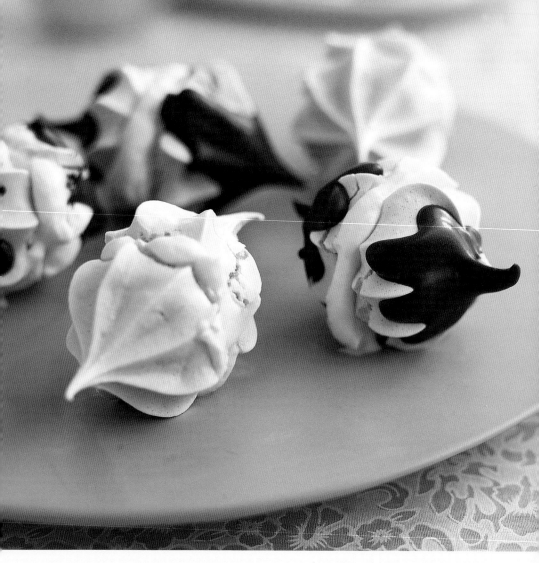

THESE LITTLE GEMS ARE GREAT
FOR PARTIES AND CERTAINLY
DON'T FEEL LIKE SPECIAL DIET
FOOD. THE MERINGUE KISSES CAN
BE DIPPED IN MELTED CHOCOLATE
OR CAROB OR JOINED TOGETHER
WITH WHIPPED CREAM. THEY'RE
SURE TO IMPRESS.

nutrition per meringue: Energy 31 Cal
Fat 0 g
Saturated fat 0 g
Protein 0.3 g
Carbohydrate 7.6 g
Fiber 0 g
Cholesterol 0 mg

MERINGUE KISSES

pure maize cornstarch ^{GF}**, for dusting**
2 egg whites
⅔ cup sugar
1 tsp pure confectioners' sugar ^{GF}

PREP TIME: 20 MINUTES
COOKING TIME: 40 MINUTES
MAKES ABOUT 20

Preheat the oven to 235°F. Lightly grease two baking trays, then dust them lightly with cornstarch.

Combine the egg whites, regular sugar and a pinch of salt in the small bowl of an electric mixer. Beat on high speed for 10–12 minutes. Gently fold in the confectioners' sugar.

Spoon the meringue into a piping bag fitted with a fluted tube. Pipe stars or rosettes onto the prepared trays. Bake for about 40 minutes, or until the meringues feel firm and dry. Leave to cool in the oven with the door ajar.

HINTS:
- Make sure you use pure confectioners' sugar. Some mixtures can contain cornstarch with wheat starch in it.
- This basic meringue mixture makes small, crisp meringues that store well in an airtight container for a few days. For the best result, make sure that you have enough egg white to fully absorb the sugar.
- Once cooled, the meringue kisses can be dipped in melted gluten-free chocolate or carob. They can also be joined together with whipped cream.

BANANA LOAF

BANANA BREAD IS A REAL CROWD PLEASER AND IS DELICIOUS WARM, TOASTED OR COLD. SERVE IT FOR AFTERNOON TEA OR TOAST IT FOR A DELICIOUS BREAKFAST.

2 cups gluten-free self-rising flour
2 tsp gluten-free baking powder
⅔ cup brown sugar
¼ tsp ground cinnamon
½ cup butter, melted, cooled slightly
½ cup milk
2 eggs
3 large ripe bananas, mashed

butter, to serve
maple syrup, to serve

PREP TIME: 20 MINUTES
COOKING TIME: 50 MINUTES
SERVINGS: 8

Preheat the oven to 325°F. Grease an 8 x 4 in loaf pan. Line the base of the pan with baking paper.

Sift the flour, baking powder, sugar and cinnamon into a large bowl. In a separate bowl, whisk the butter, milk and egg together. Add the milk mixture to the dry ingredients with the mashed bananas. Use a wooden spoon to mix until well combined.

Pour the mixture into the prepared pan and smooth the surface with a spoon. Bake for 40 minutes, or until a skewer inserted into the center comes out clean. Set aside in the pan for 5 minutes before turning out onto a wire rack to cool. Serve warm or at room temperature. Cut into slices, spread with butter and drizzle with a little maple syrup.

HINTS:
- Spread the slices with a little low-fat ricotta cheese before drizzling with syrup.
- This loaf is best eaten on the day it is made.
- If you're lactose intolerant or catering for someone who is, then replace the milk with rice drink or gluten-free soy milk.
- When baking gluten-free goods, use heavy-duty pans rather than aluminium; this will help them cook evenly.

nutrition per serving: Energy 379 Cal; Fat 15.9 g; Saturated fat 9.4 g; Protein 6.1 g; Carbohydrate 51.5 g; Fiber 3.3 g; Cholesterol 89 mg

CUPCAKES

THESE SWEET LITTLE CAKES ARE READY IN A FLASH AND ARE GREAT FOR
CHILDREN'S PARTIES, ESPECIALLY WHEN DECORATED WITH GLUTEN-FREE
ICING.

½ **cup butter**
½ **cup sugar**
2 eggs, or equivalent egg replacer
1 cup gluten-free self-rising flour
½ **cup rice flour**
3 tsp gluten-free baking powder
½ **cup milk**
pure confectioners' sugar GF**, for dusting**

PREP TIME: 15 MINUTES
COOKING TIME: 20 MINUTES
MAKES 24

Preheat the oven to 350°F. Line 12 cups of two regular muffin trays with paper cases.

In the small bowl of an electric mixer, beat the butter and sugar together until light and fluffy. Add the eggs, one at a time, beating well after each addition.

Sift the dry ingredients into a large bowl. Fold the dry ingredients into the butter mixture alternately with the milk.

Spoon the mixture evenly into the muffin cups and bake for about 15–20 minutes, or until just cooked. Cool on a wire rack. Dust the cakes with pure confectioners' sugar before serving. Alternatively, leave off the confectioners' sugar and top the cakes with gluten-free icing (see below).

HINTS:
- For a dairy-free version, you can replace the butter with dairy-free margarine and the milk with gluten-free soy milk or rice drink.
- It's important to use pure confectioners' sugar to ensure no gluten has been added.
- These can be iced with carob or cocoa icing: To make the icing, sift 1½ cups pure confectioners' sugar GF and 1 tablespoon unsweetened cocoa powder GF or carob powder into a heatproof bowl. Add enough cold water to make a smooth paste. Place the bowl over a saucepan of simmering water and stir continuously until the icing softens to the required consistency.

nutrition per cake: Energy 104 Cal; Fat 5.1 g; Saturated fat 3.1 g; Protein 1.5 g; Carbohydrate 12.9 g; Fiber 0.5 g; Cholesterol 30 mg

SPONGE CAKE

4 eggs
¾ cup sugar
1 cup soy-free, gluten-free all-purpose flour, sifted
⅓ cup strawberry jam GF **(Basics)**
pure confectioners' sugar GF**, to serve**
1¼ cup whipping cream

PREP TIME: 20 MINUTES
COOKING TIME: 30 MINUTES
SERVINGS: 6—8

Preheat the oven to 350°F. Lightly grease and flour two 8 in round cake pans, then line the base with baking paper.

Beat the eggs and sugar in the small bowl of an electric mixer for about 6–7 minutes, or until light and fluffy. Very gently fold the sifted flour into the egg mixture alternately with 4 tablespoons hot water. Gently spread the mixture into the prepared pans.

Bake for about 25–30 minutes, or until lightly browned and the cakes have pulled away from the side of the pan. Turn onto a wire rack to cool.

Whip the cream into stiff peaks.

Spread the jam over the top of one sponge, and top with the cream. Place the other sponge on top and dust with confectioners' sugar.

HINTS:
- This sponge has no wheat flour and no chemical raising agent, but relies on air for its lightness. Take great care when folding in dry ingredients. Use a large slotted metal spoon to ensure light, even folding.
- If you prefer, you can use apricot, peach or pear jam instead of strawberry.
- Since some confectioners' sugar mixtures contain gluten, it's important to use pure confectioners' sugar.
- If you are lactose intolerant, you can make mock whipped cream. To make the mock whipped cream, sprinkle 1 teaspoon powdered gelatin over 4 tablespoons cold water in a small heatproof bowl. Stand the bowl in a small saucepan of simmering water and stir until the gelatin has dissolved. Cool slightly. Beat ½ cup dairy-free margarine, 3 tablespoons sugar and ½ teaspoon natural vanilla extract in a small bowl with electric beaters until pale in color. Gradually add the cooled gelatin mixture and beat until light and fluffy.

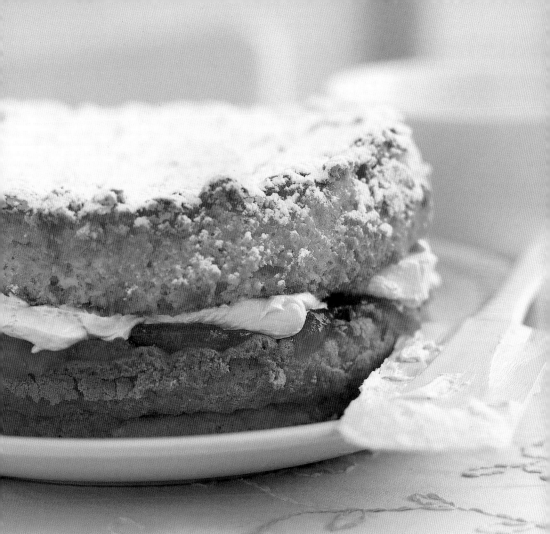

GLUTEN-FREE COOKING HAS
COME A LONG WAY. IT USED TO
BE REALLY DIFFICULT TO MAKE
A LIGHT, FLUFFY GLUTEN-FREE
SPONGE, BUT NOW YOU CAN
EASILY MAKE ONE AT HOME
USING A GOOD QUALITY
GLUTEN-FREE FLOUR MIXTURE.

nutrition per serving (8): Energy 353 Cal
Fat 18.9 g
Saturated fat 11.5 g
Protein 4.3 g
Carbohydrate 42.7 g
Fiber 0.6 g
Cholesterol 123 mg

177

FLOURLESS CHOCOLATE WALNUT CAKE

THIS CAKE HAS NO FLOUR WHATSOEVER. FOR BEST RESULTS USE A PREMIUM BITTERSWEET DARK CHOCOLATE WITH A HIGH LEVEL OF COCOA SOLIDS.

1¼ cups walnuts
9 oz dark chocolate ^{GF}**, chopped**
2 tbsp whipping cream
1 tsp natural vanilla extract
½ cup sugar
6 eggs, separated
fresh raspberries, to serve
whipped cream, to serve

PREP TIME: 20 MINUTES
COOKING TIME: 40 MINUTES
SERVINGS: 8

Preheat oven to 350°F. Grease and line the base of an 8 in spring-form cake pan with baking paper.

Process the walnuts in a food processor until finely ground.

Put the chocolate, cream and vanilla extract in a heatproof bowl. Sit over a saucepan half filled with simmering water. Turn off the heat and stir the chocolate until just melted. Allow the mixture to cool a little.

Add the sugar, egg yolks and ground walnuts to the chocolate mixture and mix to combine. Using electric beaters, beat the egg whites until firm peaks form. Stir a large spoonful of the egg white into the chocolate to soften the mixture, then fold through the remaining egg white. Pour into the prepared pan. Bake for 40 minutes or until firm to touch. Leave to cool for 5 minutes, then turn out onto a wire rack to cool completely. Serve with fresh raspberries and whipped cream.

HINTS:
• Replace the ground walnuts with hazelnut meal or almond meal, if you prefer.
• You can use reduced-fat cream to help lower the fat content.

nutrition per serving: Energy 398 Cal; Fat 25.7 g; Saturated fat 8.6 g; Protein 8.7 g; Carbohydrate 34 g; Fiber 1.4 g; Cholesterol 149 mg

BIRTHDAY CAKE

A BIRTHDAY IS A SPECIAL OCCASION THAT DESERVES A TRULY SPECIAL CAKE—
LIKE THIS ONE.

pure maize cornstarch ^{GF}, **for dusting**
6 eggs
1 cup sugar
4 tbsp arrowroot
4 tbsp pure maize cornstarch ^{GF}
½ cup strawberry jam ^{GF} **(Basics)**

MARSHMALLOW FROSTING
3 tsp powdered gelatine
2¼ cups sugar

PREP TIME: 1 ½ HOURS
COOKING TIME: 45 MINUTES
SERVINGS: 10–12

Preheat the oven to 350°F. Lightly grease three 9 in round cake pans or two 11 x 7 in pans, then dust with cornstarch.

Combine the eggs and sugar in the bowl of an electric mixer. Beat until thick and light. Gently fold in the sifted arrowroot and cornstarch. Divide the mixture among the three round pans or two rectangular pans.

Bake for 25–30 minutes, or until well risen and pale golden. Turn onto wire racks to cool.

Sandwich the cooled cakes together using the jam. Place the cake on a stiff board or plate.

To make the marshmallow frosting, dissolve the gelatin in 1 cup water. Pour into a saucepan. Add 1 cup water and the sugar and mix well. Heat gently, stirring until boiling. Simmer without stirring over low heat for 15 minutes.

Remove the pan from the heat and leave to cool slightly. Scoop the frosting into the large bowl of an electric mixer and beat on high speed until the mixture doubles in bulk and becomes thick. Spread quickly over the cake, using a metal spatula.

HINT:
• Decorate the cake with your choice of gluten-free confectionery. You'll need to work quickly before the frosting sets.

nutrition per serving (12): Energy 309 Cal; Fat 2.5 g; Saturated fat 0.8 g; Protein 4 g; Carbohydrate 70.3 g; Fiber 0.2 g; Cholesterol 94 mg

179

BASICS

BEEF STOCK

about 4½ lbs beef bones

2 unpeeled carrots, chopped

2 unpeeled onions, quartered

2 tbsp tomato paste ^{GF}

2 celery stalks, leaves included, chopped

1 bouquet garni

12 black peppercorns

Preheat the oven to 415°F. Put the bones in a baking pan and bake for 30 minutes, turning occasionally. Add the carrot and onion and cook for a further 20 minutes. Allow to cool.

Put the bones, onion and carrot in a large, heavy-based saucepan. Drain the excess fat from the baking pan and pour 1 cup water into the pan. Stir to dissolve any pan juices, then add the liquid to the pan.

Add the tomato paste, celery and 10 cups water. Bring to a boil, skimming the surface as required, and then add the bouquet garni and peppercorns. Reduce the heat to low and simmer gently for 4 hours. Skim the froth from the surface regularly.

Strain through a colander, then through a fine sieve. Remove any fat from the surface. Store in the refrigerator for up to 2 days or in the freezer for up to 6 months. Makes about 8 cups.

HINT:
- To make your own bouquet garni, tie together with a string or wrap in a piece of cheesecloth (muslin) 4 sprigs parsley or chervil, 1 sprig fresh thyme and 1 bay leaf.

CHICKEN STOCK

about 4½ lbs chicken bones
2 unpeeled onions, quartered
2 unpeeled carrots, chopped
2 celery stalks, leaves included, chopped
1 bouquet garni
12 black peppercorns

Put the chicken bones, onion, carrot, celery and 14 cups water in a large, heavy-based saucepan. Bring slowly to a boil. Skim the surface as required and add the bouquet garni and peppercorns. Reduce the heat to low and simmer gently for 3 hours. Skim the froth from the surface regularly.

Strain the stock. Set aside to cool, then refrigerate until cold. Spoon off any fat that has set on the surface. Transfer to an airtight container. Store in the refrigerator for up to 2 days or in the freezer for up to 6 months. Makes about 10 cups.

HINT:
• To make your own bouquet garni, tie together with a string or wrap in a piece of cheesecloth (muslin) 4 sprigs parsley or chervil, 1 sprig fresh thyme and 1 bay leaf.

VEGETABLE STOCK

1 tbsp oil
1 onion, chopped
2 leeks, thickly sliced
4 carrots, chopped
2 parsnips, chopped

4 celery stalks, leaves included, chopped
2 bay leaves
1 bouquet garni
4 unpeeled garlic cloves
8 black peppercorns

Heat the oil in a large, heavy-based saucepan and add the onion, leek, carrot, parsnip and celery. Cover and cook for 5 minutes without coloring. Add 12 cups water. Bring to a boil. Add the bay leaves, bouquet garni, garlic and peppercorns. Reduce the heat to low and simmer for 1 hour. Skim the froth from the surface of the stock regularly.

Strain the stock. Set aside to cool, then transfer to an airtight container. Store in the refrigerator for up to 2 days or in the freezer for up to 6 months. Makes about 10 cups.

HINT:
• To make your own bouquet garni, tie together with a string or wrap in a piece of cheesecloth (muslin) 4 sprigs parsley or chervil, 1 sprig fresh thyme and 1 bay leaf.

FISH STOCK

about 4½ lbs chopped fish bones, heads and tails
1 celery stalk, leaves included, roughly chopped
1 onion, chopped
1 unpeeled carrot, chopped
1 leek, sliced
1 bouquet garni
12 black peppercorns

Place the fish bones, celery, onion, carrot, leek and 8 cups of water in a large, heavy based saucepan. Bring slowly to a boil. Skim the surface as required and add the bouquet garni and peppercorns. Reduce the heat to low and simmer very gently for 20 minutes. Skim off any froth regularly.

Ladle the stock in batches into a sieve lined with damp muslin sitting over a bowl. To keep a clear fish stock, do not press the solids, but simply allow the stock to strain undisturbed. Allow to cool, then store in the refrigerator for up to 2 days, or in the freezer for up to 6 months. Makes about 6 cups.

FRENCH DRESSING (VINAIGRETTE)

3 tbsp olive oil
2 tbsp white wine vinegar

1 tsp wholegrain mustard
freshly ground pepper, to taste

Place all the ingredients in a small screw-top jar and shake well. Use immediately. Makes about ½ cup.

ITALIAN DRESSING

3 tbsp white wine vinegar
3 tbsp olive oil

½ tsp sugar
1 tbsp chopped fresh basil

Put the vinegar, olive oil and sugar in a bowl and whisk to combine. Stir in the basil and leave to stand for 15 minutes before serving. Makes about ½ cup.

MAYONNAISE

2 egg yolks
¼ tsp salt
1 cup canola oil
½ tsp lemon juice

Put the egg yolks and salt in a bowl and whisk together until well combined and thick.

Gradually whisk in the oil, drop by drop, from a teaspoon until a quarter of the oil has been added. The mixture should be thick at this stage. Very slowly pour in the remaining oil in a thick steady stream, while continuing to beat steadily. Beat in the lemon juice. Store in a glass jar in the refrigerator for up to 3 days. Makes about 1 cup.

HINT:
- Mayonnaise can be made in a blender or food processor. Use the same ingredients as above. Blend the eggs and salt for a few seconds. With the motor running, pour in the oil in a steady thin stream. When all the oil has been added, the mixture should be thick.

MANGO CHUTNEY

1 tbsp oil
2 garlic cloves, crushed
1 tsp grated ginger
2 cinnamon sticks
4 cloves
½ tsp chilli powder

2 large (about 2 lbs) fresh or frozen ripe mango flesh, roughly chopped
1½ cups white vinegar
1 heaping cup sugar

Heat the oil in a heavy-based saucepan over medium heat, add the garlic and ginger and fry for 1 minute. Add the remaining ingredients and bring to a boil.

Reduce the heat to low and cook for 1 hour, or until the mango is thick and pulpy, like jam. It should fall in sheets off the spoon when it is ready. Add salt, to taste, and more chilli if you wish. Remove the whole spices.

Pour the chutney into hot sterilized jars (wash the jars in boiling water and dry them thoroughly in a warm oven). Seal the jars and allow to cool completely. Store in a cool place or in the refrigerator after opening. Makes about 2 cups.

BASIC TOMATO SAUCE

5–6 (about 3½ lbs) tomatoes
1 tbsp olive oil
1 onion, finely chopped
2 garlic cloves, crushed
2 tbsp tomato paste GF
1 tsp dried oregano
1 tsp dried basil
1 tsp sugar

Score a cross on the base of each tomato, place in a bowl of boiling water for 10 seconds, then plunge into cold water and peel away the skin from the cross. Finely chop the flesh.

Heat the oil in a saucepan. Add the onion and cook, stirring, over medium heat for 3 minutes, or until soft. Add the garlic and cook for 1 minute. Add the tomato, tomato paste, oregano, basil and sugar. Bring to a boil, then reduce the heat and simmer for 20 minutes, or until the sauce has thickened slightly. Store in an airtight container in the refrigerator for up to 2 days or in the freezer for up to 6 months. Makes about 6 cups.

STRAWBERRY JAM

6 cups sugar
3½ lbs strawberries
½ cup lemon juice

Warm the sugar by spreading in a large baking dish and heating in an oven preheated to 235°F for 10 minutes, stirring occasionally. Put two plates in the freezer. Hull the strawberries and put in a large pan with the lemon juice, sugar and ½ cup water. Warm gently, without boiling, stirring carefully with a wooden spoon. Try not to break up the fruit too much.

Increase the heat and without boiling, continue stirring for 10 minutes, until the sugar has thoroughly dissolved. Increase the heat and boil, without stirring, for 20 minutes. Start testing for the setting point: place a little jam on one of the cold plates, a skin will form on the surface and the jam will wrinkle when pushed with a finger. It could take up to 40 minutes to reach setting point. Remove from the heat and leave for 5 minutes before removing any scum that forms on the surface. Pour into hot sterilized jars, seal and label. Makes about 4 cups.

SHORTCRUST PASTRY

1¼ cups gluten-free, all-purpose flour
6 tbsp cold butter, chopped
1 egg, lightly beaten

FOOD PROCESSOR METHOD. Put the flour and butter in a food processor and pulse until crumb-like. Add the egg and 1–2 teaspoons water until the dough is starting to come together. Don't add any more water than necessary. Turn out onto a surface lightly dusted with gluten-free flour and knead briefly to bring together the dough into a smooth ball. Wrap in plastic wrap and refrigerate to firm. Knead the dough well to help the dough hold together. Roll out between two sheets of baking paper that have been lightly dusted with gluten-free flour until large enough to line the prepared pan or dish. Refrigerate the lined dish for 30 minutes to prevent shrinkage and cracking.

BOWL METHOD. Sift the flour into a large bowl. Rub the butter into the flour with your fingertips until the mixture resembles dry breadcrumbs. Make a well in the center and add the egg and 1–2 teaspoons water until the dough is starting to come together. Don't add any more water than necessary. Turn out onto a a surface lightly dusted with gluten-free flour and knead briefly to bring together the dough into a smooth ball. Wrap in plastic wrap and refrigerate to firm. Roll out between two sheets of baking paper that have been lightly dusted with gluten-free flour until large enough to line the prepared pan or dish. Refrigerate the lined dish for 30 minutes to prevent shrinkage and cracking.

HINTS:
- This pastry is very thin and is more difficult to handle than pastry that contains gluten. It is soft and malleable so when lining the dish, fill any tears and cracks, if necessary.
- You can use margarine to make the pastry if you prefer. It will need a little less water, if any. The pastry is softer and harder to handle, but firms enough when refrigerated.
- A combination of gluten-free flours usually produces a better pastry than using only one type of flour. This is why many commercial gluten-free flour mixes contain a number of different flours.
- Sometimes gluten-free baked goods don't work because the oven is not working properly. You can check whether your oven is working properly by using an oven thermometer, which can be purchased from a good kitchenware shop.

SWEET SHORTCRUST PASTRY

1¼ cups gluten-free, all-purpose flour
3 tbsp confectioners' sugar GF
6 tbsp cold butter, chopped
1 egg, lightly beaten

FOOD PROCESSOR METHOD. Put the flour and sugar in a food processor and briefly pulse to combine. Add the butter and pulse until crumb-like. Add the egg and 1–2 teaspoons water until the dough is starting to come together. Don't add any more water than necessary. Turn out onto a surface lightly dusted with gluten-free flour and knead briefly to bring together the dough into a smooth ball. Wrap in plastic wrap and refrigerate to firm. Knead the dough well to help the dough hold together. Roll out between two sheets of baking paper that have been lightly dusted with gluten-free flour until large enough to line the prepared pan or dish. Refrigerate the lined dish for 30 minutes to prevent shrinkage and cracking.

BOWL METHOD. Sift the flour and confectioners' sugar into a large bowl. Rub the butter into the flour with your fingertips until the mixture resembles dry breadcrumbs. Make a well in the center and add the egg and 1–2 teaspoons water until the dough is starting to come together. Don't add any more water than necessary. Turn out onto a surface lightly dusted with gluten-free flour and knead briefly to bring together the dough into a smooth ball. Wrap in plastic wrap and refrigerate to firm. Roll out between two sheets of baking paper that have been lightly dusted with gluten-free flour until large enough to line the prepared pan or dish. Refrigerate the lined dish for 30 minutes to prevent shrinkage and cracking.

HINTS:
- The pastry is more difficult to handle than pastry that contains gluten. It is soft and malleable so when lining the dish, just fill any tears and cracks, if necessary.
- You can use margarine to make the pastry. It will need a little less water, if any. The pastry is softer and harder to handle, but firms enough when refrigerated.
- A combination of gluten-free flours usually produces a better pastry than using only one type of flour. This is why many commercial gluten-free flour mixes contain a number of different flours.

Contact information for celiac/dermatitis herpetiformis support groups

USA
Celiac Disease Foundation
13251 Ventura Boulevard, #1
Studio City, CA 91604
Phone: 818 990 2354
Email: cdf@celiac.org
Internet: www.celiac.org

CANADA
Canadian Celiac Association
5170 Dixie Road, Suite 204
Mississauga, ON L4W 1E3
Phone: 905 507 6208
Email: info@celiac.ca
Internet: www.celiac.ca

AUSTRALIA
The Coeliac Society of Australia
First Floor, 306 Victoria Avenue
Chatswood, NSW, 2067
Phone: 02 9411 4100
Email: info@coeliac.org.au
Internet: www.coeliac.org.au

GREAT BRITAIN
Coeliac UK
Suites A-D Octagon Court
High Wycombe, Bucks HP11 2HS
Phone: 01494 437 278
Internet: www.coeliac.co.uk

NEW ZEALAND
Coeliac Society of New Zealand Inc.
PO Box 35 724
Browns Bay
Auckland 1330
Phone: 09 820 5157
Email: coeliac@xtra.co.nz
Internet: www.coeliac.co.nz

191